PORRIDGE
& Muesli

PAVILION

VIOLA ADAMSSON | PHOTOGRAPHS BY BRUNO EHRS | DESIGN BY LISA KULLBERG

THANKS TO PROFESSOR TOMMY CEDERHOLM FOR FACT-CHECKING

First published in the United Kingdom in 2015 by
Pavilion
1 Gower Street
London
WC1E 6HD

ISBN 978-1-910496-29-9

A CIP catalogue record for this book is available from the British Library.

10 9 8 7 6 5 4 3 2 1

Reproduction by Mission Productions Ltd, Hong Kong
Printed by Toppan Leefung Printing Ltd, China

This book can be ordered direct from the publisher at www.pavilionbooks.com

TEXT AND RECIPES: Viola Adamsson
PHOTOGRAPHY: Bruno Ehrs
STYLIST: Liselotte Forslin
ASSISTANT: Nora Nordlund
DESIGN: Lisa Kullberg
PROJECT MANAGER: Ingela Holm
EDITOR: Gunilla Wagner

The publisher would like to thank Frida Green for her work on this book.

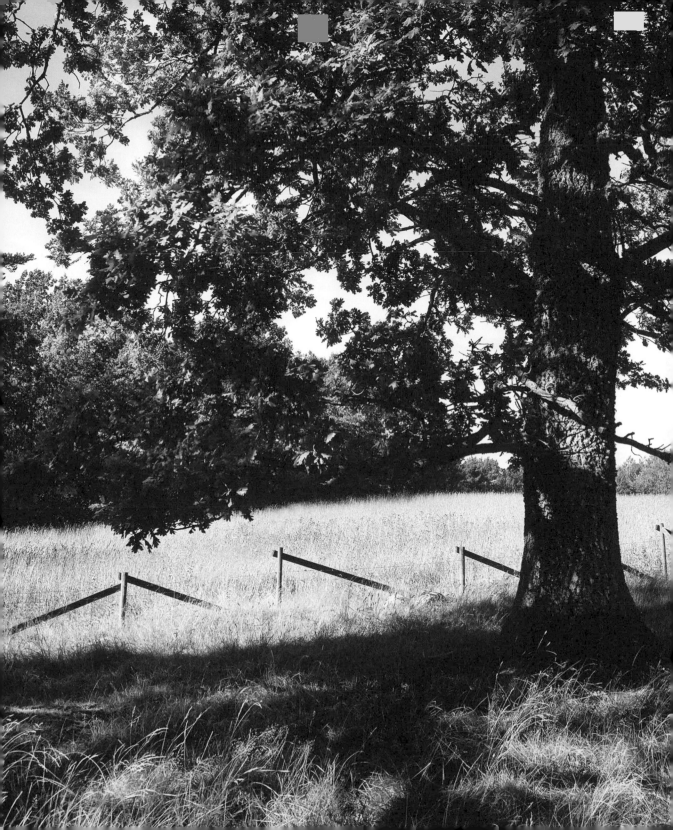

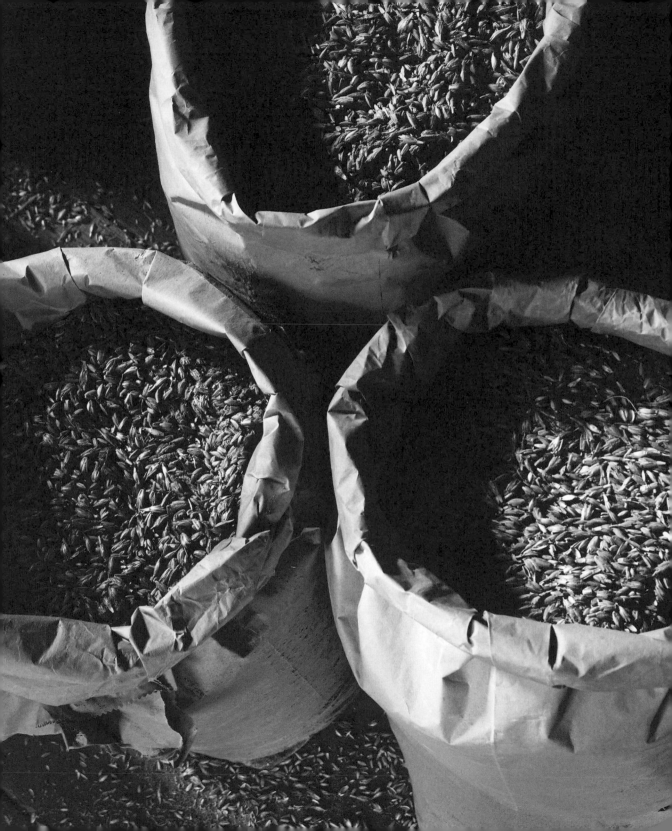

CONTENTS

SIMPLE AND INGENIOUS 6

PORRIDGE MEMORIES 7

OAT PORRIDGE RECIPES 8

BARLEY PORRIDGE RECIPES 16

CEREAL GRAINS 20

THE NUTRITIONAL VALUES OF PORRIDGE 22

WHAT CAN YOU USE TO MAKE PORRIDGE? 25

COOKING PORRIDGE 26

RYE PORRIDGE RECIPES 28

WHEAT PORRIDGE RECIPES 30

NUTRITIOUS PORRIDGE TOPPINGS 38

DIFFERENT PORRIDGE RECIPES 42

PORRIDGE BREAD RECIPES 74

MUESLI AND GRANOLA RECIPES 80

FRUIT AND JAM RECIPES 86

NUTRITIONAL DATA 94

RECIPE INDEX 96

SIMPLE AND INGENIOUS

Some flour, flakes or grains, water and perhaps some salt, a pan, whisk or spoon and, hey presto, you've got a meal. Porridge is right on trend – it has become a healthy alternative to other fast food in our modern urban culture and is now frequenting the menus of chic cafés and restaurants.

While the term 'fast food' usually has negative connotations, porridge really is a healthy fast food. Plus it can be combined with many healthy accompaniments. You can even avoid washing a pan if you use a microwave, although I do think porridge cooked in a pan tastes different from porridge cooked in a microwave. It could have something to do with the slower heating (my own speculation). Anyway there are tricks for cleaning the porridge pan (see page 26).

Porridge is a simple way to get both whole grains and dietary fibre into your diet. National recommendations for dietary fibre intake vary, but the consensus is that we should be eating around 30g/1oz per day, while the recommended daily intake of whole grains is around 75g/3oz (per 2400 calories) per day. One portion of rolled-oat porridge provides 4g/⅛oz of dietary fibre and 40g/1½oz of whole-grain ingredients while a portion of porridge made from rye will supply 8g/¼oz of dietary fibre and 40g/1½oz whole-grain ingredients. Doctor W's Healthy Porridge (see page 54) will give you about 14g/½oz of dietary fibre in a single portion!

The filling factor

Porridge lines the stomach so effectively that many people fill up on porridge and last all day long. Others may experience a 'hole in the stomach' – that is, they get hungry after a portion of porridge. I belong in that category. You have to keep on trying and find the variety of porridge that suits you best. I find that rye flakes mixed in with the rolled oats makes the porridge more filling.

The consistency of porridge depends on your cooking method and also the choice of whole, cut or chopped grains, flakes and flour. A whisked porridge will be smoother than a stirred one. Classic whisked porridges include Rye Flour Porridge (see page 28) and Wheat Flour Porridge with Butter (see page 30). Stirred porridges include Oat Porridge (see page 8) and Rye Flake Porridge (see page 28). Black, grey, brown and smooth porridge are old names for Rye Flour Porridge (see page 28) and Barley Porridge with Oats (see page 17) cooked with water. Black and White Porridge (see page 58) was traditionally made with milk, wheat flour, rice grains or semolina.

During the 18th century, porridge and gruel were often served several times a day, especially as 'evening porridge'. Porridge for breakfast is an early 20th-century invention, while various different types of porridge have always been served on festive occasions, such as weddings and harvest.

Popularity of different grains tends to be regional and affected by the local crops. Only in the 18th century did rice-grain porridge become part of the peasants' diet as a festive food.

PORRIDGE MEMORIES

When it comes to porridge, everyone has an opinion – even those who are trying interesting combinations for the first time and have no preconceptions about how porridge should be served. A good example is the porridge combination I saw in Falun during the Nordic World Cross-Country Ski Championship in 1993, where we tried Japanese oat porridge with crisp fried bacon – not easy to eat with chopsticks! Bacon with oat porridge isn't completely unconventional – not that long ago Swedish woodcutters ate fried back bacon with their porridge, and cross-country skiing burns just as many calories. I also remember from the same championship that Norwegian cross-county skiers topped their porridge with Brunost – their delicious caramelized brown cheese.

Another porridge served with fried back bacon – and lingonberry jam – is *nävgröt*, a festive Swedish classic made from toasted oat flour and served as a lunch dish. I learnt from a coach for the Swedish skiing team that you should be relaxed about cooking *nävgröt*, just bring water to the boil, add the oat flour, then stir occasionally. Unlike whisked porridge, this should be lumpy and dry so it is easy to transport for lunch. A similar rye or barley porridge is *motto* or *mutti*. We can partly thank King Karl IX for the introduction of *nävgröt* and *mutti* to Sweden, as he invited Finnish settlers to come and live in the desolate forests in order to cut them down and cultivate the land, and it was the Finns who brought these dishes to Sweden.

In 1988 I was in the US and saw on the news that oats could help to lower slightly increased cholesterol levels, primarily oat bran. I had not heard of oat bran in Sweden before, so I went on a shopping expedition to several supermarkets in Detroit to buy some, but it was sold out everywhere. In one hour, the people of Detroit had all gone out to buy oat bran. I got hold of some a few days later and since then I have eaten delicious oat bran porridge every morning. Plenty of research now confirms its cholesterol-lowering qualities.

OAT PORRIDGE

Porridge made from rolled oats is the classic recipe, but there are several different types of rolled oats to choose from. Larger oat flakes will be ready in 3 minutes, porridge oats and thinner flakes will be ready in 2 minutes. Those who are gluten intolerant can still enjoy porridge if they use gluten-free rolled oats.

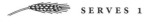 **SERVES 1**

100G/3½OZ/1 CUP ROLLED OATS
250ML/9FL OZ/GENEROUS 1 CUP WATER
½–1 PINCH OF SALT
TO SERVE, SEE BELOW

Put the rolled oats and water in a pan and add the salt. Bring to the boil, then leave to simmer for about 3 minutes, stirring occasionally so that the porridge doesn't stick to the base of the pan. If you stir the oat flakes into boiling water, you'll get a grainier porridge with more character.

Milk and Apple Sauce (see page 93) are the classic accompaniments. Also try serving the porridge with yogurt and raspberries, or soured cream, cinnamon and sugar. Serve with Brunost (caramelized whey cheese) and strawberry jam, and you've got a Norwegian classic.

Tip To cook in the microwave, mix together the oats, water and salt in a bowl. Microwave on Medium for about 3 minutes, then stir well.

OAT PORRIDGE WITH CARAMEL COATING – SERVES 2 >>>

2 PORTIONS OAT PORRIDGE (SEE ABOVE)
2 TBSP SUGAR

If you don't have a blow torch, preheat the grill to high. Cook the porridge according to the recipe, then divide between two heatproof bowls. Sift the sugar over the bowls and caramelize using a culinary blow torch or under the grill until the sugar has melted into a golden caramel. This may take 5–6 minutes.

Try topping the porridge with fresh fruit, such as sliced bananas, strawberries, raspberries and blueberries.

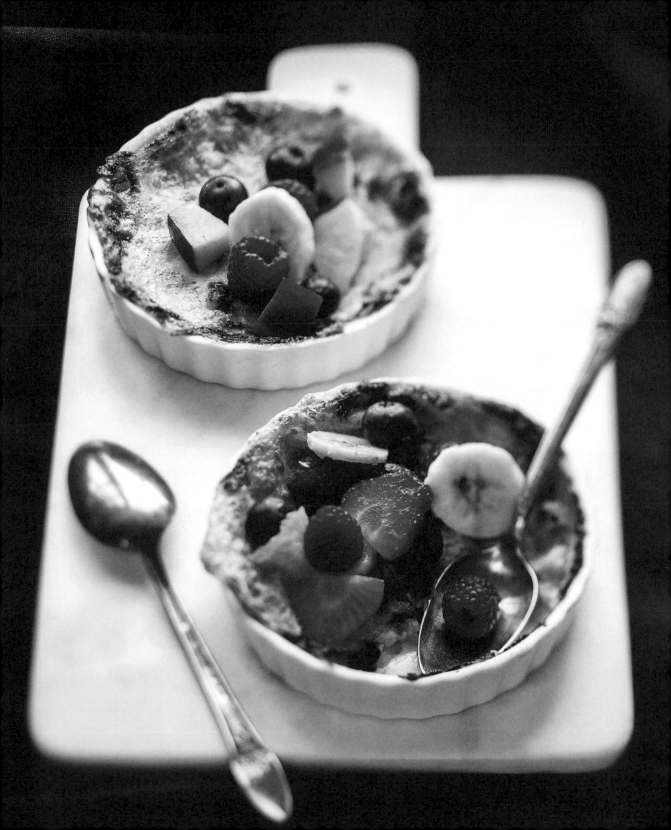

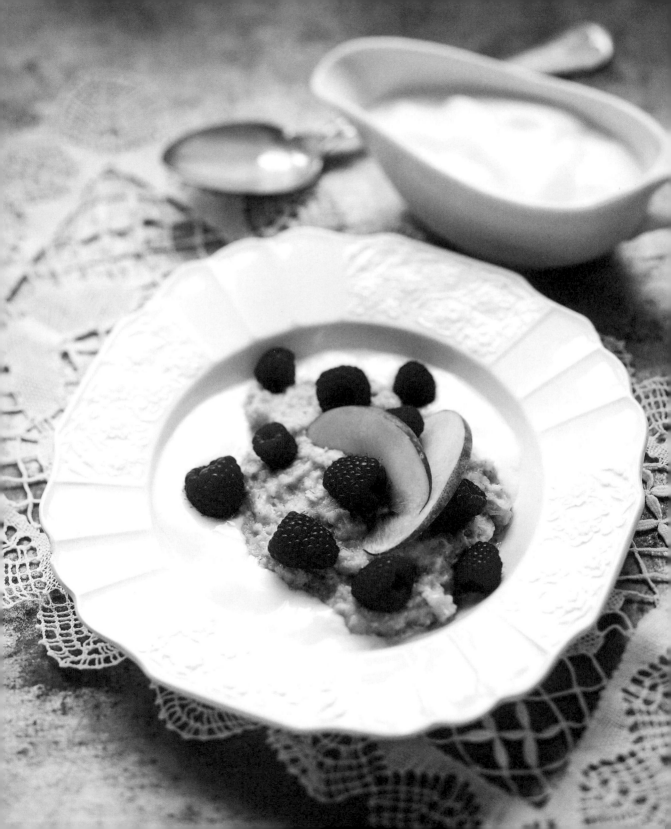

OAT PORRIDGE MELBA

This oat porridge takes its inspiration from the classic dessert, Peach Melba. Consisting of vanilla ice cream, peaches and raspberries, it is named after Dame Nellie Melba, who was an Australian soprano singer. When the vanilla ice cream is replaced with oat porridge, it is transformed into a new and exciting dish.

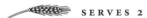 **SERVES 2**

2 PORTIONS OAT PORRIDGE (SEE PAGE 8)
100G/3½OZ/¾ CUP RASPBERRIES, CRUSHED
2 FRESH NECTARINES OR PEACHES, STONED AND SLICED
VANILLA YOGURT, TO SERVE (OPTIONAL)

Cook the porridge according to the recipe and divide between two bowls. Top with the raspberries and sliced nectarines or peaches.

Serve with vanilla yogurt, if you like.

Tip You could use drained, tinned peaches in fruit juice instead of the nectarines.

OAT BRAN PORRIDGE

If you eat porridge regularly, the nutrients it contains can help to reduce slightly increased cholesterol levels. One portion of porridge made with oat bran or two portions made from rolled oats contain the amount of beta-glucan needed for lowering cholesterol.

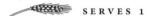 SERVES 1

250ML/9FL OZ/GENEROUS 1 CUP WATER
40G/1½OZ/SCANT ½ CUP OAT BRAN
½–1 PINCH OF SALT
A KNOB OF BENECOL OR OTHER CHOLESTEROL-LOWERING SPREAD
BLUEBERRY PURÉE

Mix together the water, oat bran and salt in a pan. Bring to the boil, then cover and simmer for 3–4 minutes, stirring occasionally, until thick.

Serve with a dollop of Benecol and a spoonful of blueberry purée.

Tip To cook in the microwave, mix the water, oat bran and salt straight onto a deep bowl. Microwave on Medium for 3–4 minutes. Stir before serving.

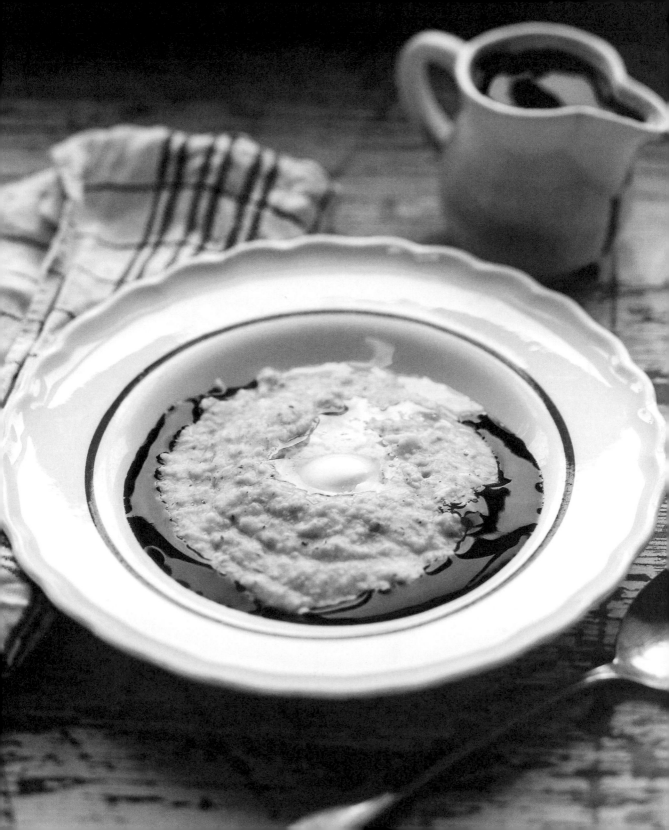

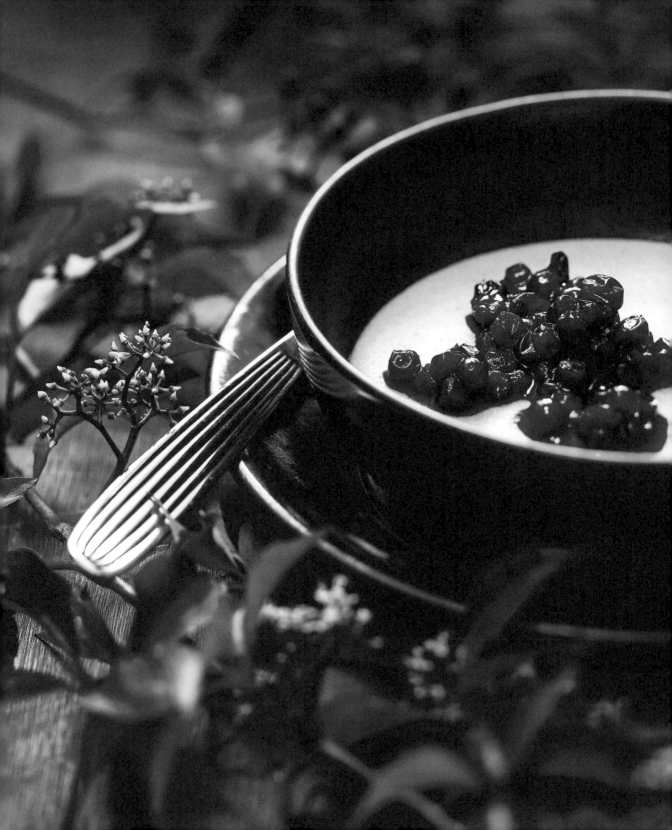

TOASTED OAT FLOUR PORRIDGE

This flour is made from soaked, toasted and ground oats. In the soaking process, the minerals in the oats become more easy to absorb. In Sweden, this would be served with lingonberry jam.

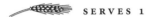 **SERVES 1**

250ML/9FL OZ/GENEROUS 1 CUP WATER OR MILK
30G/1OZ/¼ CUP OAT FLOUR, TOASTED
½ PINCH OF SALT
CRANBERRY JAM, MILK OR YOGURT, TO SERVE

Mix together the water or milk, flour and salt in a pan. Bring to the boil, then continue to simmer over a low heat for 3–5 minutes, stirring constantly.

Serve with cranberry jam, milk or yogurt.

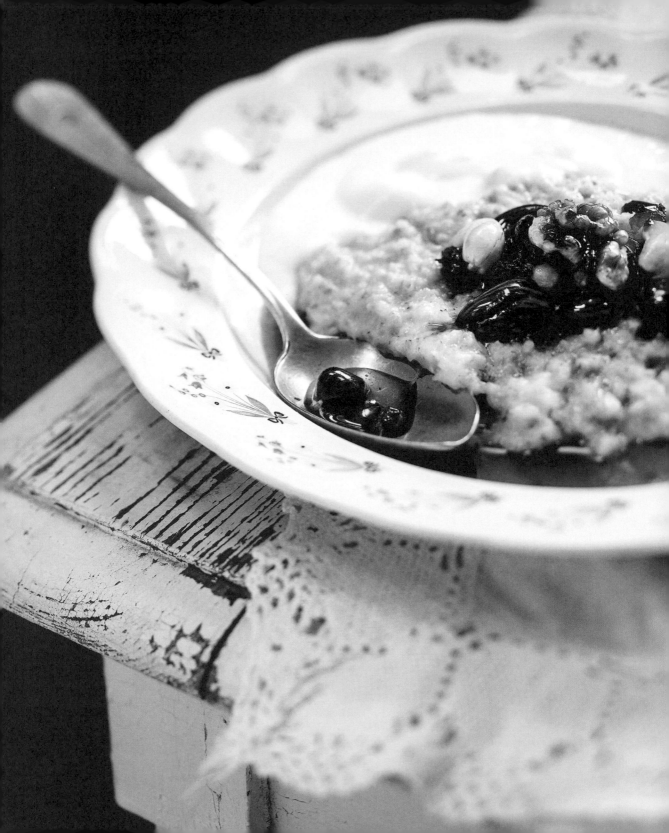

BARLEY PORRIDGE WITH OATS

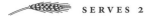 **SERVES 2**

70G/2½OZ/SCANT ½ CUP WHOLEMEAL BARLEY GRITS
500ML/17FL OZ/GENEROUS 2 CUPS WATER
½ PINCH OF SALT
200ML/7FL OZ/SCANT 1 CUP WATER OR MILK
40G/1½OZ/SCANT ½ CUP ROLLED OATS WITH WHEATBRAN
MIXED NUTS, HONEY AND VANILLA YOGURT, TO SERVE

Mix together the wholemeal barley grits, water and salt in a heavy-based or non-stick pan. Bring to the boil, then lower the heat, cover and simmer for about 35 minutes until the grits have softened. Stir occasionally to ensure the mixture doesn't stick to the base of the pan.

Add the water or milk and the rolled oats. Return to the boil and simmer for 3–5 minutes, stirring constantly.

Scatter with mixed nuts, drizzle with honey and serve with vanilla yogurt.

CHRISTMAS PORRIDGE WITH WHOLEMEAL GRITS

Porridge made from wholemeal barley grits used to be served at festive occasions. When the rice grain was introduced to the Scandinavian peasantry in the 18th century, the barley grits were mixed with rice grains in the porridge pan. Grits from hulled barley are wholemeal and contribute to a slow and steady rise in blood sugar levels. Barley contains the soluble fibre beta-glucan.

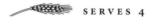 SERVES 4

60G/2¼OZ/SCANT ⅓ CUP PUDDING RICE
50G/1¾OZ/⅓ CUP WHOLEMEAL BARLEY GRITS
300ML/½ PINT/GENEROUS 1¼ CUPS WATER
½ TSP SALT
700ML/1¼ PINTS/3 CUPS WHOLE MILK
2 CINNAMON STICKS
GROUND CINNAMON, SUGAR AND MILK OR APPLE SAUCE (SEE PAGE 93) AND MILK, TO SERVE

Put the pudding rice, wholemeal barley grits, water and salt in a large pan. Bring to the boil, then cover and simmer over a low heat for about 10 minutes, stirring occasionally.

Add the milk and cinnamon sticks and stir well. Return to the boil, then simmer gently over a very low heat for 40 minutes, without stirring, until the grits are soft. If the porridge is too thin, remove the lid and simmer it for an extra few minutes, stirring.

Sprinkle with ground cinnamon and sugar and serve with milk as a traditional Christmas porridge, or serve with apple sauce and milk.

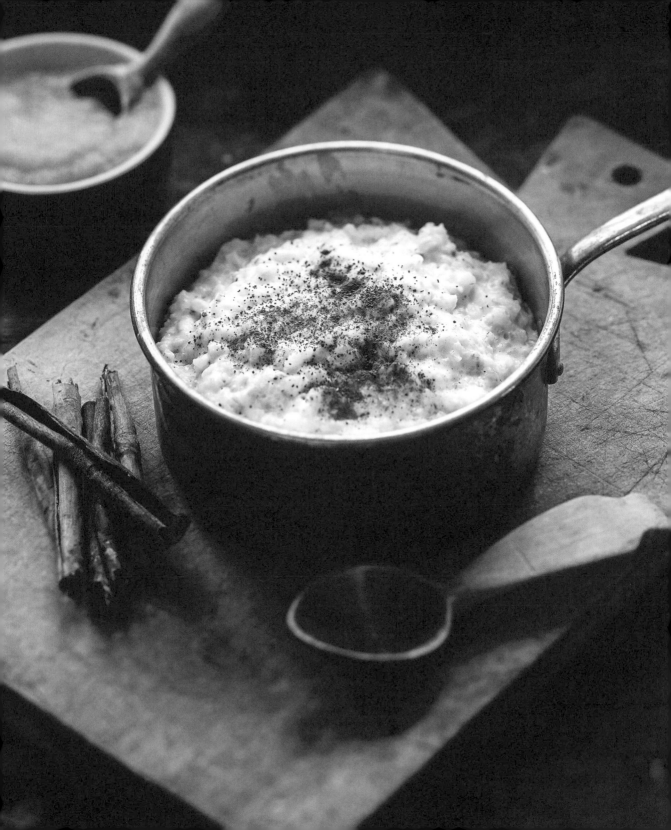

CEREAL GRAINS

Oats

Oats are now the grain most commonly used for porridge. Interest in including oats in the diet for health reasons has continued to rise, especially as the beneficial effects of oats on cholesterol levels in the blood and maintaining blood sugar levels have been confirmed by the European Food Safety Authority, EFSA.

In comparison to wheat and barley, oats contain more fat and more complete protein. The fat is mostly unsaturated.

From oat grains, rolled oats, oat bran, oat flour, steamed oat flour, oat drink and fibre concentrate are made. There are also whole-grain oats that are used in the same way as traditional rice. Oats are gluten-free and can be eaten by those who are gluten intolerant, providing that the whole production chain, from seeds to the packaging of the finished product, is separated from other grains that contain gluten.

Barley

Along with wheat, barley is one of the oldest cultivated cereal grains and is grown all over the world. Barley is an important crop for animal food but is also used in baking, cooking and in beer and malt production.

From barley, pearl barley, barley flour, barley grits and barley flakes are produced. Barley can also be used in the same way as traditional rice.

Rye

By far the majority of the world's rye cultivation occurs between the Ural Mountains and the North Sea – having been grown in Sweden since the 13th century – so it is not surprising that cooking with rye is focused on the northern European and Scandinavian countries.

From rye, rye flour (both coarse and fine) and rye flakes are made. Almost all rye is made into flour and flakes for porridge, baking and muesli.

Wheat

Wheat is the most common cereal grain in the world. The Reverend Sylvester Graham was an early advocate of the high nutritional values of wholemeal wheat flour, hence it is sometimes still called Graham flour in the US. Wholemeal flour contains all parts of the wheat grain – the germ, endosperm and bran – so none of the nutritious qualities of the grain are lost. Other wheat flours are sifted and the bran and other elements are extracted. The extraction rate measures how much of the whole grain is used in a particular flour, starting from the centre. Wholemeal wheat flour has an extraction rate of 100 percent, while white flour made from the germ has an extraction rate of 72 percent.

Spelt is a particular type of wheat that is becoming popular because of its nutritious qualities and nutty flavour.

From wheat, different kinds of wheat flour are produced, including wholemeal wheat flour, wholemeal wheat flakes and wheat berry that is used in the same way as traditional rice.

Buckwheat

This is not actually related to wheat, but its nutritional values are similar to cereal grains. It is also gluten-free, making it particularly appealing to anyone with intolerance to other grains. It needs to be rinsed in hot water before preparing the actual porridge or, alternatively, the water can be drained off after cooking.

What is wholemeal?

As we have said, grains contain the germ, the endosperm and the bran, the outer coating that contains the most fibre, while the inside contains more starch. A wholemeal product contains all parts of the grain: that is the germ, the endosperm and the bran. Products that are 100 percent wholemeal include rolled oats, rye flour, rye flakes, wholemeal barley grits, barley flakes, barley flour and wholemeal wheat flour. Refined ingredients obviously contain a lesser percentage of the whole grain, while some products may combine refined ingredients with those that contain the full 100 percent of the grain.

THE NUTRITIONAL VALUES OF PORRIDGE

Here are some of the reasons why porridge is so popular and so good for us.

Dietary fibre

Research around the health benefits of dietary fibre took off during the 1970s when British researchers noticed a link between the quantity of faeces passed per day and the absence of typical Western diseases such as diabetes and heart and cardiovascular conditions. The average amount of faeces for those following a traditional Western diet was 100–150g/3½–5½oz per day, with motions, on average, once every three days, while for groups in Africa, whose diet contained more fibre, it was twice that, with motions three to four times a day.

Since these findings, a lot of research has been carried out to study the relationship between dietary fibre and health, and it is well documented that a diet rich in fibre has a number of benefits. It makes it easier to control one's weight, lowers the chance of developing heart and cardiovascular diseases, and lowers the chance of developing metabolic syndrome, type 2 diabetes and some forms of cancer.

Dietary fibre increases the sensation of being full and therefore make it less likely that we over-eat, thus contributing to weight loss. And whether or not weight loss happens, dietary fibre tends to reduce inflammation in the body. A part of dietary fibre's effect on inflammation is thought to be linked to the short-chain fatty acids that are produced in the large intestine when dietary fibre and bacteria meet. When this happens, a fermentation process is started in the large intestine, which means that the dietary fibre is broken up and new compounds – short-chain fatty acids, such as acetic acid, propionic acid and butyric acid – are produced. The short-chain fatty acids lower the pH value in the large intestine, are absorbed by the blood stream and have an effect on the metabolism and possibly on inflammation in the body.

One side effect of eating a lot of dietary fibre is the production of gases such as carbon dioxide, hydrogen gas and methane gas, which can result in flatulence, but the choice between flatulence and heart disease, cancer or high blood pressure is a no-brainer. In any event, once your body gets used to a high-fibre diet, the problem should diminish.

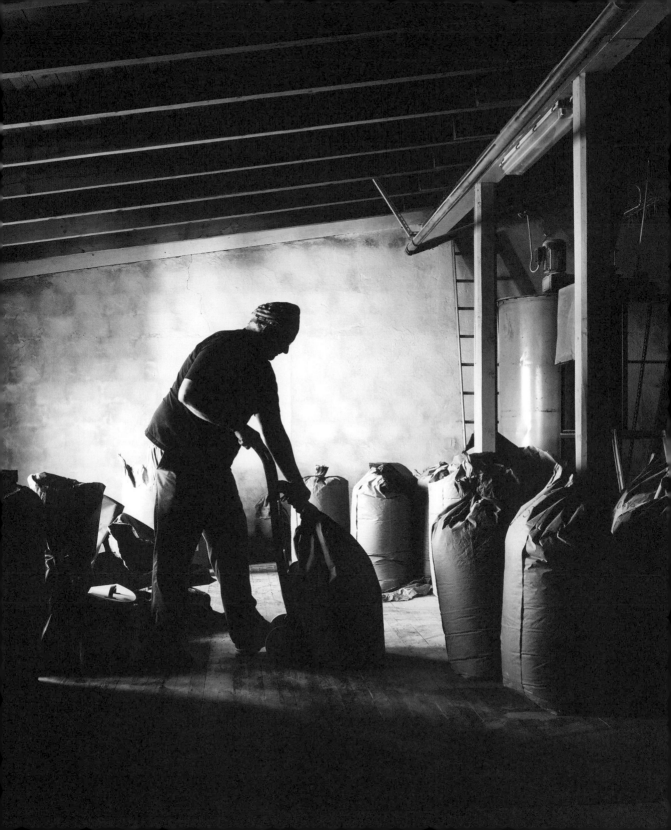

Wholemeal porridge

Many long-term health benefits that are attributed to a fibre-rich diet could come from different components or qualities of wholemeal products – not just from dietary fibre.

Wholemeal grains contain soluble and insoluble dietary fibre, but they also contain vitamins, minerals and other bioactive compounds. The bran, or the skin, contains soluble and insoluble dietary fibre, B vitamins and minerals such as magnesium, iron, zinc and manganese. The germ contains about 25 percent fat, most of it unsaturated, vitamin E, B vitamins and plant sterols.

Depending on which wholemeal product you use for making porridge, the end product will score a different glycaemic index, or GI number. A porridge that is cooked from whole, pinhead or cut groats – for example, Barley Porridge with Oats (see page 17), will score a lower GI than a porridge cooked from flour, flakes or rolled oats.

Type of porridge, fibre and health effects

Cereal grains contain different types of dietary fibre and vary when it comes to nutritional content. Because of this, it is good to vary or use a mixture of whole, pinhead or cut or cracked grains, flour, grits and flakes from rye, barley, oat and wheat in the same porridge to profit from the different health benefits of each grain.

Oat and barley contain a special kind of soluble dietary fibre, beta-glucan, which helps to lower harmful cholesterol (LDL) without lowering the good cholesterol (HDL). The fibre beta-glucan traps bile salts and transports them out of the body in the natural way. To produce new bile salts, the body uses cholesterol from the blood, resulting in an overall reduction in the amount of cholesterol in the body. One portion of Oat Bran Porridge (see page 12) contains the 3g of beta-glucan needed for lowering cholesterol by 5–10 percent. Oat porridge and barley porridge contain 1–1½g of beta-glucan per portion.

Dietary fibre can also have a positive effect on blood-sugar levels. The blood-sugar levels will rise more slowly after a meal rich in dietary fibre and, in particular, rich in soluble dietary fibre, something that is good for everyone and especially important for those suffering from diabetes.

Rye is regarded as being more filling than other cereal grains. One reason for this could be that rye contains more dietary fibre in total than other grains. There are both soluble and insoluble dietary fibres in rye. The insoluble dietary fibres prevent constipation while the soluble dietary fibres, beta-glucan and arabinoxylan, contribute to lowered cholesterol levels. Rye contributes to a better regulation in blood-sugar levels, especially as the rye fibre has a lower insulin requirement in comparison to wheat. One simple way to eat more rye is to cook porridge from rye flour and rye flakes or to mix rye flakes into your muesli.

Most of the dietary fibre in wholemeal wheat is insoluble and prevents constipation by giving more volume to the contents in the intestine and therefore shortening the time waste products remain in the body.

Porridge and GI

Porridges cooked from wholemeal flour, grits or flakes have one thing in common: they all contain high-quality carbohydrates, that is, they contain both wholemeal and dietary fibre. The glycaemic index (GI) of porridge varies and is dependent on, among other things, whether or not the porridge has been made from whole and pinhead/cut groats. The thickness of the flakes and grits that the porridge is made from also has an effect on the GI. Porridge cooked from thick flakes, grits and whole groats has a lower GI than porridge cooked from flour or thinner flakes, as the starch becomes less accessible for the digestive fluids to get to in thicker flakes.

The amount of soluble dietary fibre also has an effect on porridge's GI. Porridge cooked from oat and barley is richest in soluble dietary fibre and can therefore contain a slightly lower GI. When porridge cools down, the starch becomes retrograded, and it behaves like dietary fibre in the body. Fried porridge contains a lot of retrograded starch and has a lower GI in comparison to the same kind of freshly cooked porridge.

WHAT CAN YOU USE TO MAKE PORRIDGE?

FLAKES is a name for cereal products from rye, oat, corn, barley and wheat that have been pre-treated with steam and heat and then rolled.

FLOUR is made from the finely ground grains of various cereals. When the endosperm, bran and germ are all included, it is a wholemeal flour. In sifted flour, bran and germ have been removed.

GRITS AND CUT GROATS are peeled, partly chopped or hulled and polished grains. A grit is between a groat and flour particle in size.

OAT BRAN is what you get when the outer, fibre-rich part of the grain (the bran) is shaved off.

WHEAT GERMS are the germs from wheat grains.

WHOLE GRAINS (kernels) from oats, rye, barley and wheat can be mixed with flour, flakes, grits and cut groats, and soaked overnight to shorten the cooking time.

COOKING PORRIDGE

On the stove

To make a whisked porridge, you need a heavy-based or non-stick saucepan and a whisk. Bring the water to the boil, then sprinkle in the oatmeal while whisking constantly so you get a smooth and lump-free porridge. You'll improve with practice as it is considered an art to make an expertly whisked, smooth rye-flour porridge.

For a stirred porridge, you need a similar heavy-based or non-stick pan and a wooden spoon or fork. Add the flakes or grits to cold water in the pan, bring to a boil, stirring occasionally, then continue to stir occasionally as it cooks. Flakes and grits can also be placed in boiling water, then you get a thicker porridge with more texture.

In the microwave

Mix the flakes or grits with cold water and a little salt, if you wish, directly on a serving dish to make a single portion, or in a larger bowl for more servings, and stir. Set the microwave to Medium and microwave the porridge for 3–4 minutes, stirring occasionally.

Washing the pans

For an ordinary porridge pan, fill the pan with cold water to cover all the porridge residue, then leave it to stand for at least an hour. Scrape off the remnants using a dishwashing brush or a soft dough scraper before washing the pan.

If the porridge has burnt in the pan, first scrape off as much as possible, then pour some washing up liquid into the pan, fill with warm water and leave to stand for at least an hour. Scrape off the burnt porridge with a dough scraper, then wash the pan. You may need to repeat the process for badly burnt pans.

ALTERNATIVE INGREDIENTS

If you replace the water or milk in your porridge with other liquids, the porridge will take on a quite different character. Try rosehip syrup, blueberry purée or oat milk. Or you could try yogurt, soya or almond milk, fruit and berry coulis, sauce or even jam.

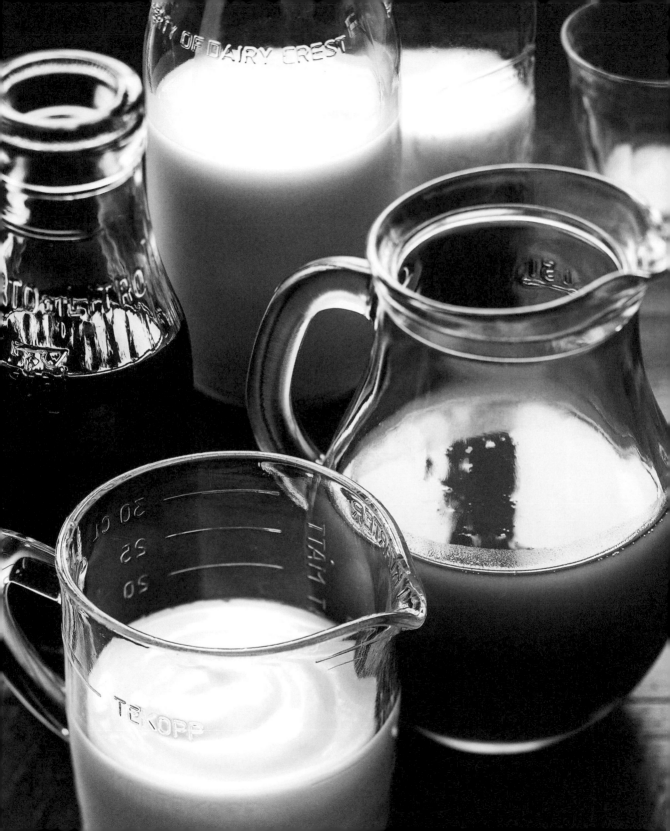

RYE FLOUR PORRIDGE

A classic whisked porridge made with water, rye-flour porridge is generally considered to be more filling than other types of porridge. Rye flour is 100 percent wholemeal regardless of whether you use fine or coarse flour.

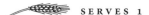 **SERVES 1**

250ML/9FL OZ/GENEROUS 1 CUP WATER
½–1 PINCH OF SALT
40G/1½OZ/½ CUP RYE FLOUR, FINE OR COARSE
FRESH FIGS, QUARTERED, WALNUTS AND FRUIT YOGURT, TO SERVE

Bring the water and salt to the boil, then whisk in the flour. Cover and leave to simmer gently over a low heat for 8–10 minutes until thick, stirring occasionally so that the porridge doesn't stick to the base of the pan.

Serve with fresh figs, walnuts and fruit yogurt.

RYE FLAKE PORRIDGE

Rye flakes are also 100 percent wholemeal. Rye contains almost equal amounts of soluble and insoluble dietary fibre. Wholemeal rye kick-starts digestion but also has the ability, like oats, to lower cholesterol levels in the blood.

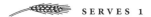 **SERVES 1**

40G/1½OZ/HEAPED ⅓ CUP RYE FLAKES
1 TSP LINSEEDS
250ML/9FL OZ/GENEROUS 1 CUP WATER
½–1 PINCH OF SALT
FRESH STRAWBERRIES, MILK OR VANILLA YOGURT, TO SERVE

Mix together the rye flakes, linseeds, water and salt in a pan. Bring to the boil, then simmer for about 5 minutes, stirring occasionally. Serve with fresh strawberries and milk or vanilla yogurt.

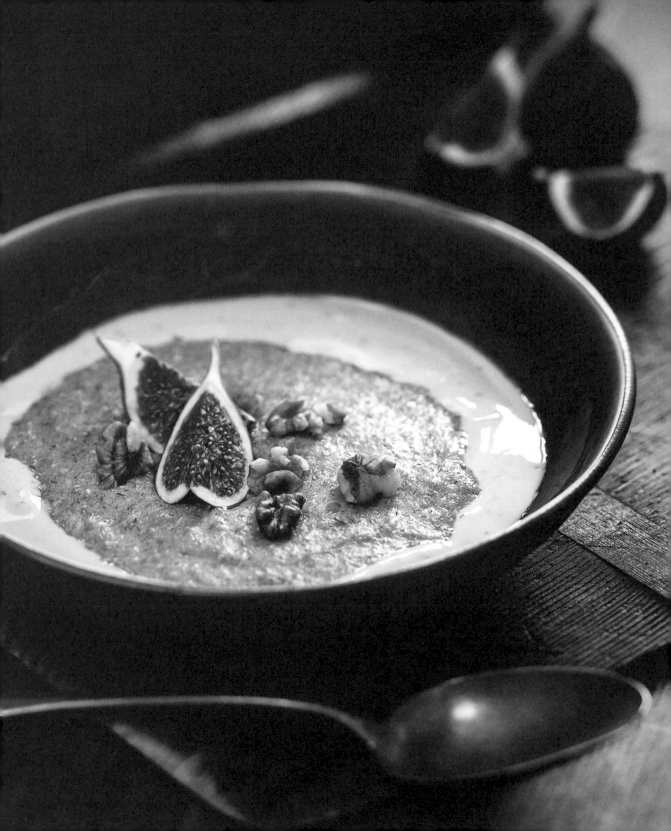

WHEAT FLOUR PORRIDGE WITH BUTTER

The finished porridge has a silky smooth texture. Leave a small dollop of butter to melt in the hot porridge. Wheat-flour porridge provides 1g of dietary fibre per portion.

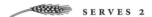 **SERVES 2**

50G/1¾OZ/HEAPED 1⅔ CUPS PLAIN WHEAT FLOUR
400ML/14FL OZ/1¾ CUPS WHOLE MILK
1 PINCH OF SALT
1 PINCH OF SUGAR
2 KNOBS OF BUTTER
COLD MILK, TO SERVE

Mix the flour with a little of the milk in a small bowl to make a smooth paste. Bring the remaining milk to the boil in a heavy-based pan.

Whisk the flour and milk mixture into the boiling milk, then simmer for 3–5 minutes over a low heat, stirring occasionally. Season with salt and sugar.

Put a knob of butter into each bowl and leave it to melt into the porridge, then serve with cold milk.

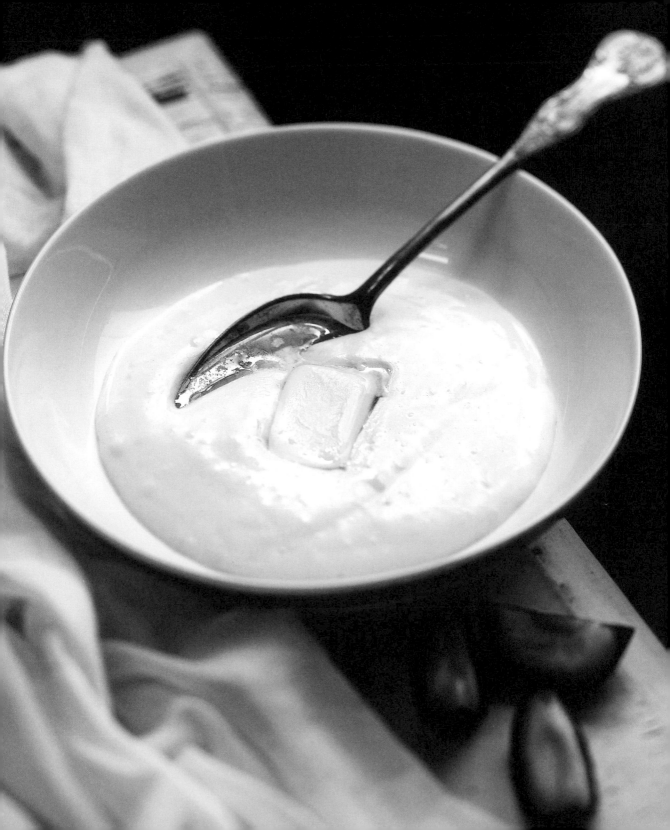

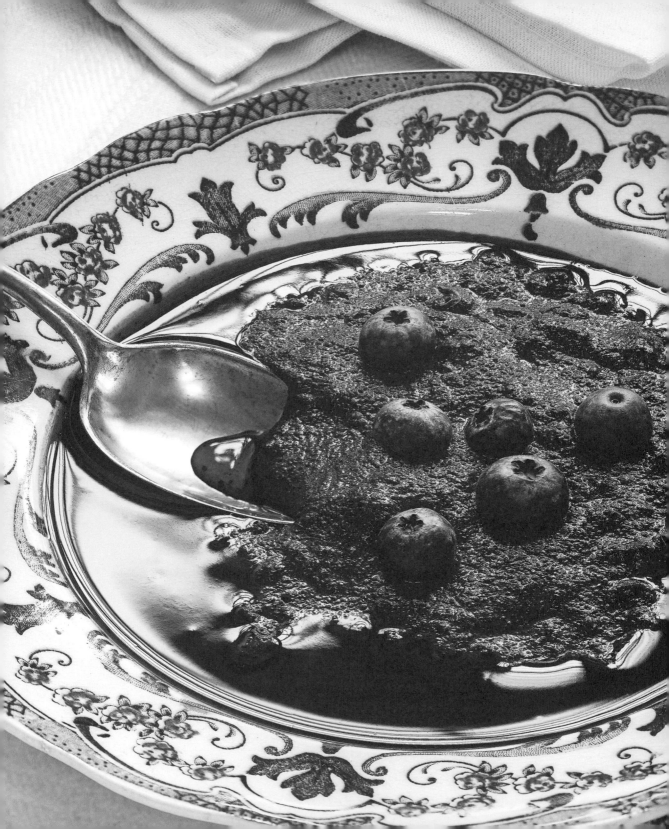

BLUEBERRY PORRIDGE

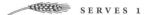 SERVES 1

50G/1¾OZ/HEAPED ⅓ CUP BLUEBERRIES, PLUS EXTRA TO SERVE
150–200ML/5–7FL OZ/⅔–SCANT 1 CUP MILK
1 TBSP SUGAR
½ PINCH OF SALT
2 TBSP SEMOLINA OR WHOLEMEAL WHEAT GRITS
BLUEBERRY COULIS, TO SERVE

Mix together the blueberries, milk, sugar and salt in a pan and bring to the boil. Remove the pan from the heat and whisk in the semolina or wholemeal wheat grits. Return to the hob, cover and simmer over a low heat for about 5 minutes until thick. Stir occasionally so that the porridge doesn't get stuck to the base of the pan. Serve with blueberry coulis and fresh blueberries.

CRÈME FRAÎCHE PORRIDGE

This is a Norwegian speciality called rømmegrøt, *which is traditionally made with a local, high-fat soured cream (*rømme*). If you are lucky enough to get hold of some, you can use it instead of the crème fraîche.*

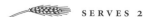 SERVES 2

100ML/3½FL OZ/SCANT 1 CUP CRÈME FRAÎCHE
ABOUT 40G/1¾OZ/⅓ CUP PLAIN FLOUR, SIFTED
ABOUT 300ML/½ PINT/GENEROUS 1¼ CUPS WHOLE MILK
1 PINCH OF SALT
SUGAR AND GROUND CINNAMON, TO SERVE

Put the crème fraîche in a heavy-based pan over a very low heat, cover and simmer very gently for about 15 minutes. It should not boil. Stir one-third of the flour into the pan to make a smooth porridge. Continue to simmer gently until the fat starts to separate. Skim off the fat but save it for serving.

Add the rest of the flour into the pan and stir into a smooth porridge. Bring to a simmer for 1–2 minutes while stirring constantly. Season with salt to taste. Serve with the skimmed fat, sugar and cinnamon.

BLUEBERRY AND RASPBERRY PORRIDGE

In Scandinavia, any porridge made with blueberries and raspberries is called Queen Porridge.

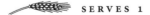 SERVES 1

60G/2¼OZ/½ CUP BLUEBERRIES AND RASPBERRIES, PLUS EXTRA TO SERVE
150–200ML/5–7FL OZ/⅔–SCANT 1 CUP MILK, PLUS EXTRA TO SERVE
½–1 TBSP SUGAR
½ PINCH OF SALT
2 TBSP SEMOLINA OR WHOLEMEAL WHEAT GRITS

Bring the blueberries, raspberries, 150ml/5fl oz/⅔ cup of the milk, the sugar and salt to the boil in a small pan. Remove the pan from the heat and whisk in the semolina or wheat grits. Return the pan to the heat, cover and simmer over a low heat for about 5 minutes until thick. Stir occasionally so that the porridge doesn't stick and add the remaining milk, if necessary. Serve with raspberries, blueberries and cold milk.

SEMOLINA PORRIDGE

Semolina is milled from the centre of durum wheat grain.

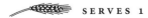 SERVES 1

1 TSP BUTTER OR MARGARINE
200ML/7FL OZ/SCANT 1 CUP WHOLE MILK
2 TBSP SEMOLINA
½ TBSP SUGAR
½–1 PINCH OF SALT
RAISINS OR PRUNES (OPTIONAL)
RASPBERRIES AND MILK OR MIXED FRUIT AND BERRY COULIS, TO SERVE

Melt the butter in a pan over a low heat. Add the milk and bring to the boil. Remove from the heat and whisk in the semolina, sugar and salt. Add the raisins or prunes, if using. Cover and simmer for 5 minutes over a low heat. Serve either warm or cold with fresh raspberries and milk, or mixed fruit and berry coulis.

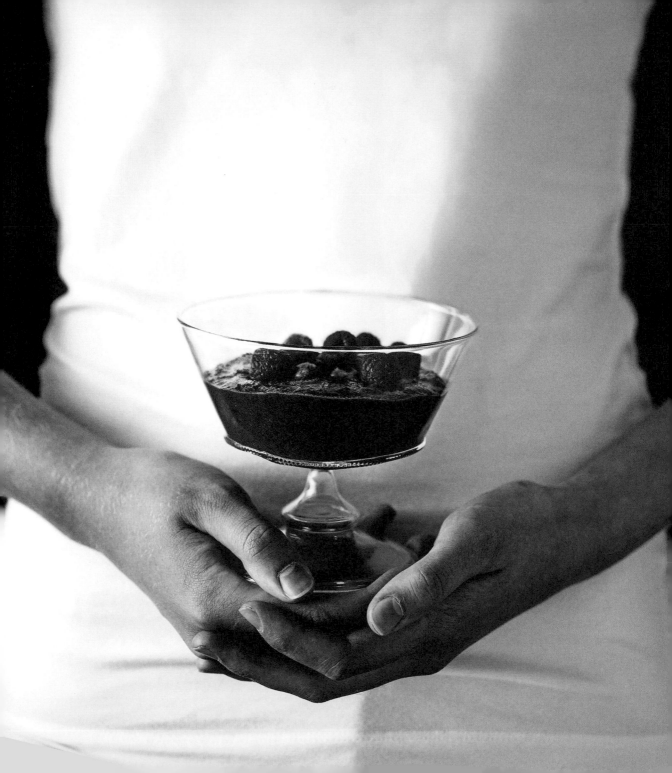

WHOLEMEAL WHEAT PORRIDGE

Another name for this recipe is Graham porridge, after the Reverend Sylvester Graham who was a dietary reformer in 19th-century America. He campaigned for a strict diet based on wholewheat flour, fresh vegetables and fruit. This version is a little less austere than the original!

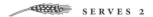 SERVES 2

250ML/9FL OZ/GENEROUS 1 CUP MILK
250ML/9FL OZ/GENEROUS 1 CUP WATER
1 PINCH OF SALT
WHOLEMEAL WHEAT GRITS (GRAHAM GRITS)
APPLE AND PSYLLIUM SEEDS OR COLD MILK, GROUND CINNAMON, SUGAR AND JAM, TO SERVE

Bring the milk, water and salt to the boil in a heavy-based pan. Whisk in the wholemeal wheat grits and bring back to the boil, stirring continuously. Simmer the porridge over a low heat for 5 minutes, stirring occasionally so that it doesn't stick to the base of the pan.

Serve with apple and psyllium seeds or cold milk, ground cinnamon, sugar and jam.

Tip To make in a microwave, mix together the milk, water and salt in a bowl. Microwave on High for about 2 minutes. Whisk in the wholemeal wheat grits. Microwave on Medium for 2 minutes, stir the porridge, then continue to cook on Medium for about 5 minutes. Stir and serve.

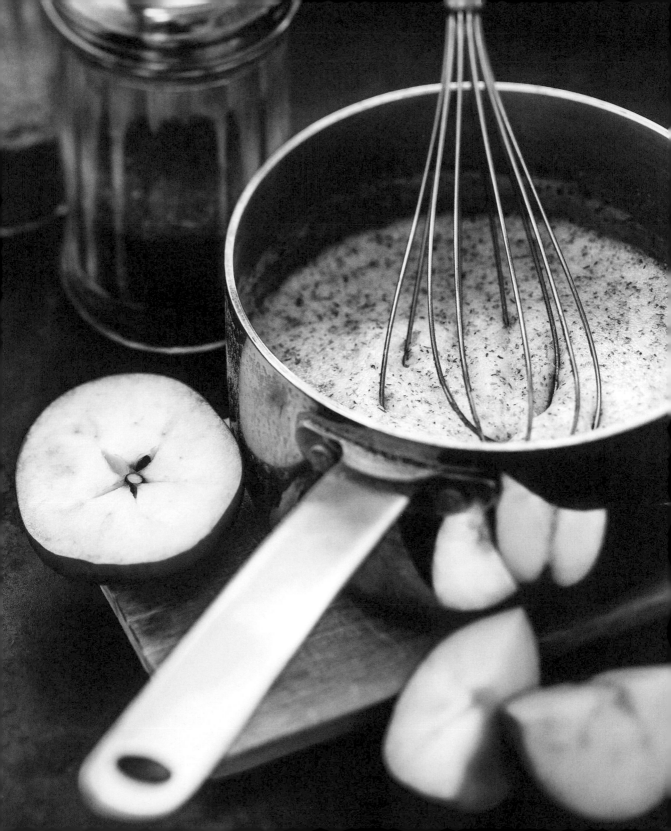

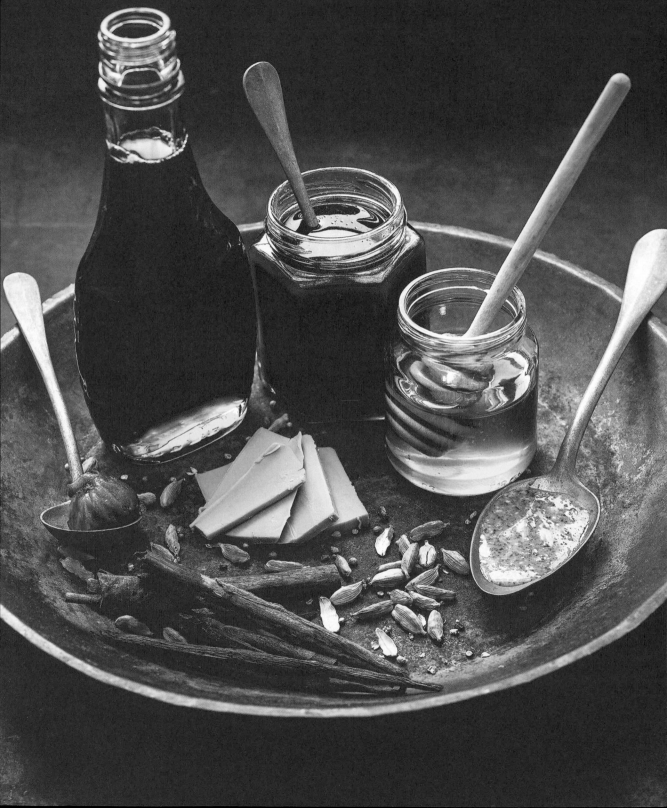

NUTRITIOUS PORRIDGE TOPPINGS

There are so many delicious ingredients that you can add to your porridge. Here are a few ideas – let your imagination run riot!

Fresh fruit and berries

Pears, apples and plums contain many beneficial vitamins, minerals and antioxidants as well as a significant amount of vitamin C, flavonoids and dietary fibre.

Fresh berries are great too. In the Nordic countries, we tend to use rosehips, blueberries, blackcurrants, gooseberries, strawberries, raspberries, blackberries, cranberries, lingonberries, cloudberries and sea-buckthorn. Apart from the last three, these are readily available to most people and they all have one thing in common – they are rich in vitamin C, folate and potassium.

The most colourful berries are rich in other kinds of antioxidants, as well as vitamin C, and in a number of other bioactive compounds. There are several positive health effects linked to deep colours in fruit and berries, with blueberries being the standalone winner! Blueberries contain anthocyanin, a flavonoid as well as a very strong colourant with antioxidant qualities. In the US, blueberries are sometimes called brainberries, because they are regarded as having a positive effect on the vessels in the brain. Blueberries are also good for the eyesight. There is a difference between the blueberries that grow wild in the forest and the ones that are cultivated. A sure sign that you are eating the best blueberries is that your mouth turns blue. Strawberries are a good source of folate, while blackcurrants and redcurrants are rich in potassium. Cloudberries, a Scandinavian speciality, are rich in vitamin C.

Dried fruit and nuts

Drying fruit and berries is a traditional way to preserve the summer and autumn harvests. Apples, plums, pears, cherries, figs, raisins, apricots and rosehips are common fruits for drying. After the drying process, the amount of vitamin C decreases while other vitamins, minerals and antioxidants become more concentrated. The level of dietary fibre is also high in dried fruit and berries.

Nuts

Almonds, and other nuts, have been used since pre-historic times by several civilizations as a part of the diet due to their nutritional content but also as a medicine to cure and treat illnesses. The Greeks used them to cure the common cold and for digestive problems, but also as an aphrodisiac. The almond is thought to have been the first domesticated tree in the Middle East.

About 50g/1¾oz of nuts per day, especially almonds, hazelnuts and walnuts, will help to lower harmful cholesterol and improve the relationship between bad and good cholesterol.

Almonds and other nuts are a source of monounsaturated fat and the essential polyunsaturated fatty acids, linoleic and alpha-linoleic acid. Nuts also contain plant sterols, which could be the substance that helps to lower the cholesterol in the blood.

Seeds

Psyllium and linseed are two examples of mucilage-producing plants. Linseeds should be eaten whole, as when crushed, harmful substances (cyanide) are made accessible for the body to absorb. One to two tablespoons of whole linseeds a day to treat constipation is regarded as risk-free.

Psyllium seeds – also known as ispaghula and isabgol – are small, shiny, brown seeds from the *Plantago ovata* plant, which grows wild and under cultivation in the Mediterranean and India. The seeds swell in water into a mucilaginous gel, and they have traditionally been used to treat constipation, but research shows that 6g of psyllium seeds per day also helps to lower cholesterol.

Milk, soured milk and yogurt

Milk, soured milk and yogurt contribute calcium, vitamin A and D as well as B vitamins. Soured milk and yogurt have a lower lactose content than milk and can more often be tolerated by those who are sensitive to lactose. In comparison to the bacteria found in soured milk, yogurt bacteria produce more lactic acid, so yogurt has a lower lactose content than soured milk.

Honey, soft whey butter and Brunost

Honey, soft whey butter and the Norwegian caramelized cheese Brunost can be used to sweeten your porridge. Honey provides sugar (fructose and glucose) as well as small amounts of vitamins and minerals. Soft whey butter and Brunost are made from the whey that is left over from cheese production and are fortified with iron.

Nut mixture

A mix of almonds, walnuts, pine nuts, sunflower seeds and hazelnuts contributes mono- and polyunsaturated fat. Dried blueberries, cranberries and raisins contain a number of healthy bioactive substances. A mixture of nuts, dried berries and fruit combined with honey makes a nice porridge topping.

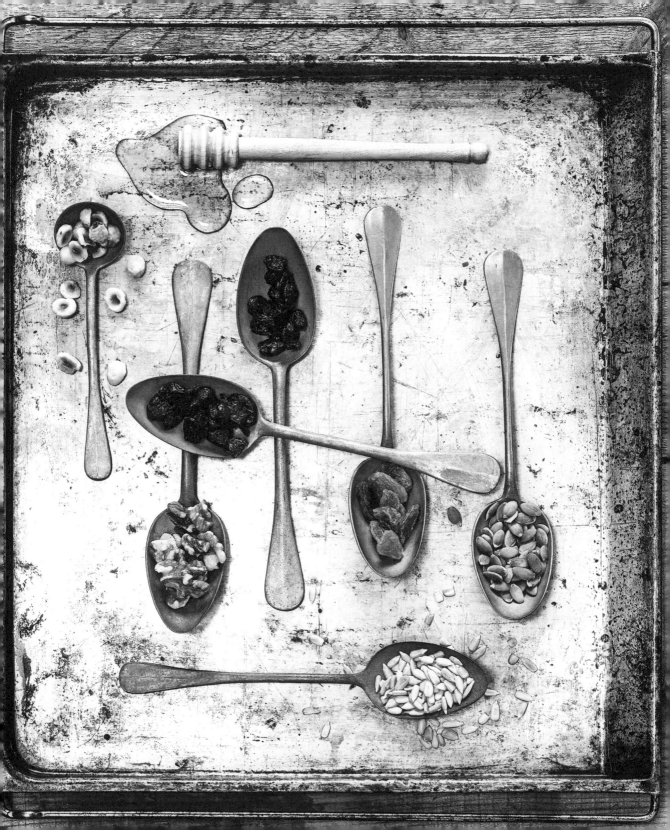

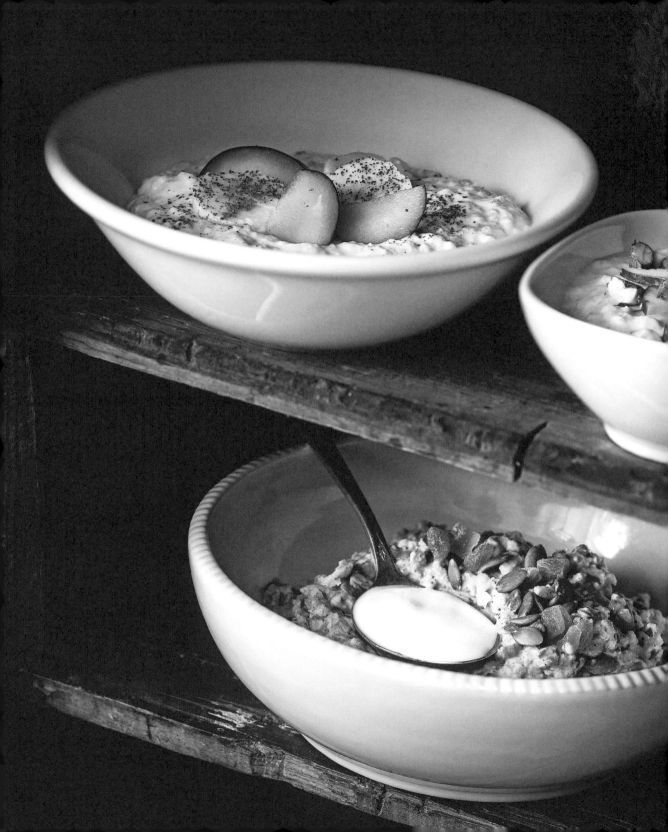

DAVOS PORRIDGE

Davos porridge is a cold porridge, great for breakfast or as an afternoon or evening snack. You can make several batches and store them in the fridge, where they will keep fresh for three days. Vary the porridge by mixing in almonds, raisins and/or prunes, then serve with fruit salad and extra yogurt.

 SERVES 1

200ML/7FL OZ/SCANT 1 CUP LOW-FAT NATURAL YOGURT WITH ½ TBSP CLEAR HONEY OR
   200ML/7FL OZ/SCANT 1 CUP VANILLA YOGURT
30G/1OZ/¼ CUP ROLLED OATS
1 TBSP RYE FLAKES, PLUMS, SLICED BANANA, GROUND CINNAMON, HONEY AND YOGURT, TO SERVE

Mix your chosen yogurt with the rolled oats and rye flakes. Leave to stand in the fridge overnight. Serve with plums, banana, cinnamon, honey and some extra yogurt.

WET MUESLI

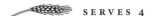 SERVES 4

100G/3¾OZ/HEAPED 1 CUP ROLLED OATS
85G/3OZ/⅔ CUP ALMONDS, COARSELY CHOPPED
60G/2¼OZ/HEAPED ⅓ CUP SUNFLOWER SEEDS
60G/2¼OZ/HEAPED ⅓ CUP PUMPKIN SEEDS
300–400ML/10–14FL OZ/1¾ CUPS ORANGE OR APPLE JUICE
1 EATING APPLE, CORED
125G/4½OZ/½ CUP VANILLA YOGURT, PLUS EXTRA TO SERVE
GROUND CINNAMON, PUMPKIN SEEDS AND CHOPPED DRIED APRICOTS, TO SERVE

Soak the rolled oats, almonds and seeds in the orange or apple juice in a bowl. Coarsely grate the apple into the oat mixture and stir well. Cover and leave to stand in the fridge overnight.

When ready to serve, mix with the yogurt and sprinkle with the cinnamon. Serve with pumpkin seeds, chopped dried apricots and some extra yogurt.

BIRCHER MUESLI

Regarded as a forerunner of naturopathy, the Swiss doctor Maximilian Bircher-Benner (1867–1939) was the creator of Bircher muesli, which is the original dish that inspired the recipes for Davos Porridge and Wet Muesli (see page 43). The recipe below is from the book The Bircher-Benner Health Guide.

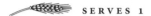 **SERVES 1**

1 TBSP ROLLED OATS

1 TBSP COLD WATER

1 TBSP LEMON JUICE

1 TBSP CREAM

1 APPLE

1 TBSP CHOPPED ALMONDS OR OTHER NUTS

Soak the rolled oats in the water overnight.

In the morning, add the lemon juice and cream. The mixture should be thicker than soup but thinner than porridge. Wash the apple and grate directly into the mixture, stirring occasionally so that the apple doesn't turn brown. Finish off by stirring in the coarsely chopped almonds or other nuts.

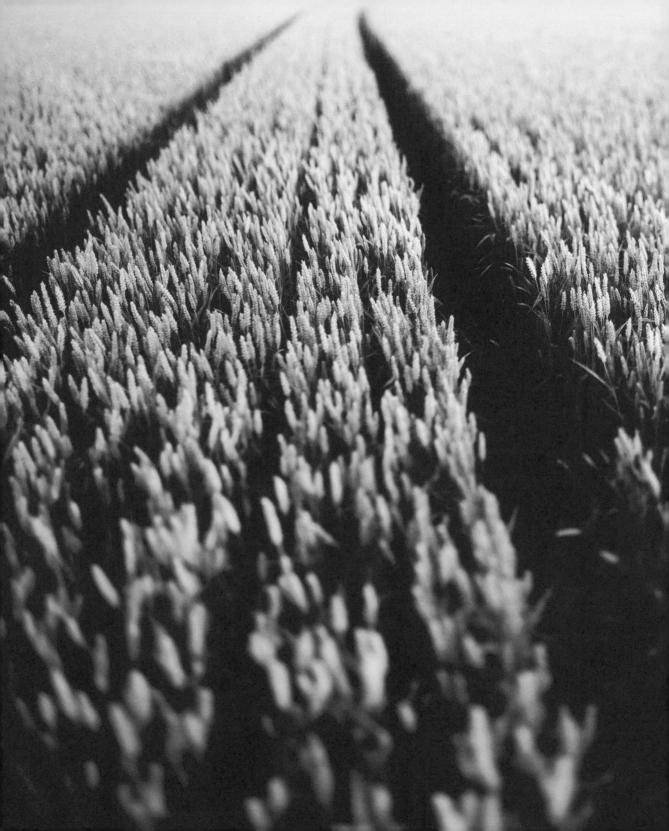

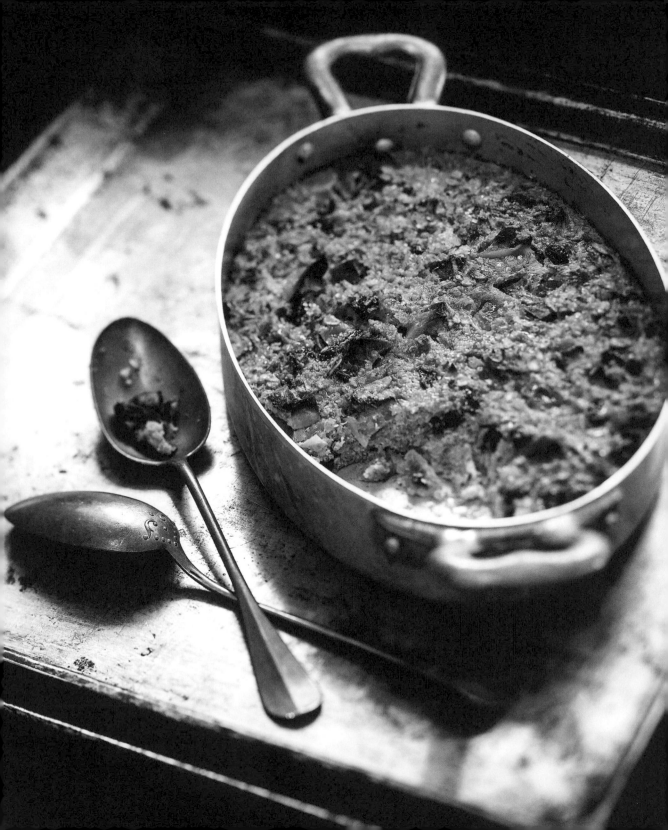

BAKED APPLE PORRIDGE

To make a perfect weekend breakfast, bake the porridge in a serving dish and take it straight to the table.

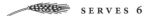 **SERVES 6**

80G/2¾OZ/HEAPED ¾ CUP SPELT FLAKES
40G/1½OZ/HEAPED ⅓ CUP QUINOA FLAKES
500ML/17FL OZ/GENEROUS 2 CUPS WHOLE MILK
2 EGGS
1 PINCH OF SALT
½ TSP FRESHLY CRUSHED CARDAMOM SEEDS
2 TBSP DEMERARA SUGAR
60G/2¼OZ/SCANT ½ CUP RAISINS
1 EATING APPLE, DICED
OIL, FOR GREASING
VANILLA YOGURT OR MILK, TO SERVE

Preheat the oven to 200°C/400°F/gas 6 and lightly grease an oven dish. Mix together the spelt and quinoa flakes with the milk, eggs and the rest of the ingredients in a bowl. Pour into the prepared dish. Bake in the middle of the oven for about 25 minutes until thick.

Serve with a dollop of vanilla yogurt or milk.

SKIER'S PORRIDGE

This porridge had its breakthrough among the Swedish national team's cross-country skiers at the World Cup in Thunder Bay, Canada in 1995. Many people find that adding rye flakes to oat porridge increases the sensation of a filling meal, making their energy last for longer. This makes two normal servings – or one if you have a skier's appetite – and would traditionally be served with lingonberry jam.

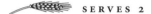 SERVES 2

60G/2¼OZ/⅔ CUP ROLLED OATS
20G/¾OZ/SCANT ½ CUP RYE FLAKES
400–450ML/14–15½FL OZ/1¾–SCANT 2 CUPS WATER
½ TSP SALT

A CHOICE OF SERVINGS
CRANBERRY JAM AND MILK
GROUND CINNAMON AND APPLE SAUCE (SEE PAGE 93)
VANILLA YOGURT

Mix the oats and rye flakes with the cold water in a heavy-based pan. Bring to the boil, then simmer the porridge for 4 minutes, stirring occasionally. Dilute with more water if it gets too thick.

Serve the porridge with classic toppings such as cranberry jam and milk. Cinnamon and apple sauce is another good combination and flavour enhancer for your porridge. Vanilla yogurt goes especially well with the rye flavour.

Tip Alternatively, you can microwave the porridge on Medium for 3 minutes.

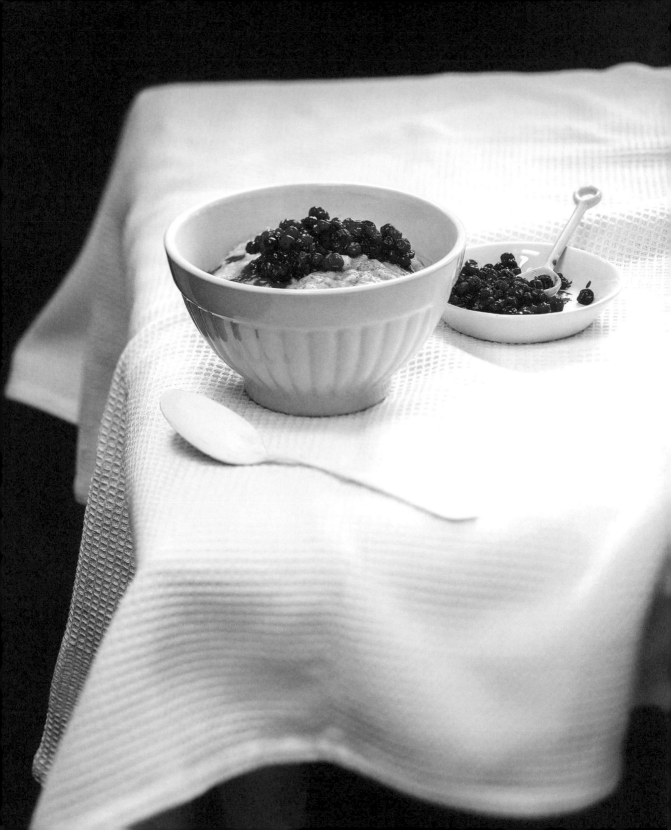

PAJALA PORRIDGE

Most healthy porridges have one thing in common – they contain a mixture of different wholemeal flakes and grits, dried fruit, bran and seeds. The mixture means that the porridge provides a whole spectrum of vitamins, minerals and other bioactive compounds, and this porridge from Pajala in Northern Sweden does exactly that.

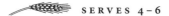 **SERVES 4–6**

4–5 STONED PRUNES
4–5 DRIED APRICOTS
30G/1OZ/SCANT ¼ CUP LINSEEDS
30G/1OZ/SCANT ¼ CUP RAISINS
½ TSP SALT
900ML–1 LITRE/1½–1¾ PINTS/3¾–4⅓ CUPS WATER
40G/1½OZ/2 TBSP OAT BRAN
80G/2¾OZ/SCANT 1 CUP ROLLED OATS WITH BRAN
RASPBERRY JAM AND MILK, OR GOOSEBERRY JAM, HONEY AND AN OAT DRINK, TO SERVE

Chop the prunes and apricots into small pieces. Mix them with the linseeds, raisins, salt and water in a stainless-steel pan. Leave to stand overnight.

The next day, add the oat bran and rolled oats. Bring to the boil, then simmer the mixture for 3–5 minutes, stirring constantly. Add a little more water if the porridge is too thick.

Serve with raspberry jam and milk, or with gooseberry jam, honey and an oat drink.

Tip Make a big batch of porridge. Quickly cool down what you don't eat straight away, then cover it and store it in the fridge for a maximum of four days. To serve, divide into portions and heat up in the microwave for a few minutes on Medium when you are ready to serve.

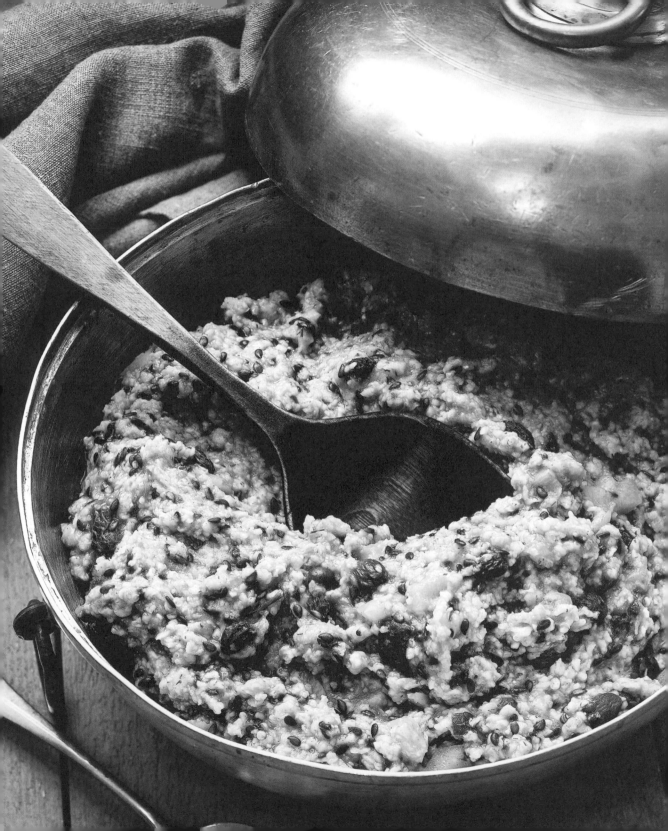

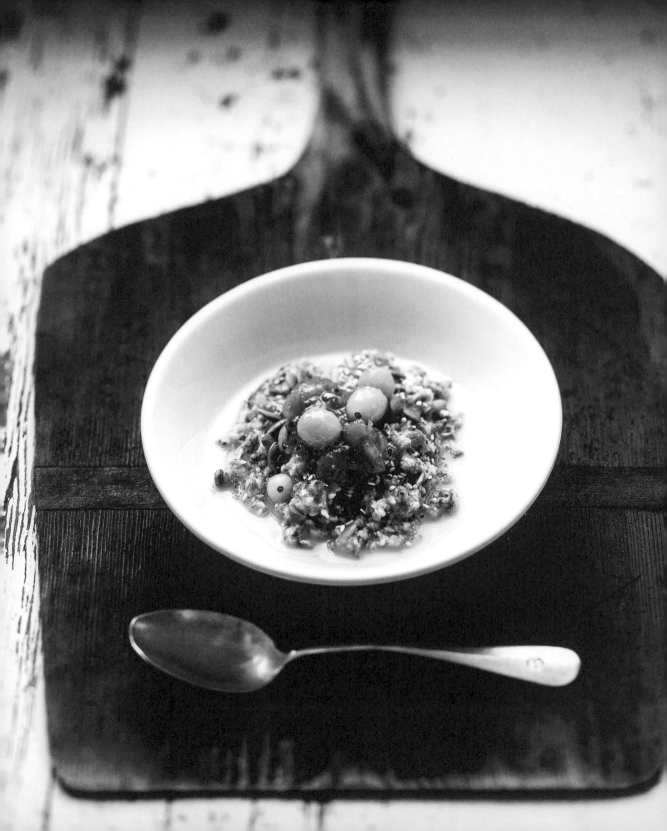

TOASTED FLAKE PORRIDGE

This mixture makes enough toasted flakes for six to eight portions, so you can make a batch and store it to use in portion sizes.

 TOASTED FLAKES – SERVES 6–8

80G/2¾OZ/SCANT 1 CUP ROLLED OATS
80G/2¾OZ/SCANT 1 CUP RYE FLAKES
80G/2¾OZ/SCANT 1 CUP SPELT FLAKES
80G/2¾OZ/SCANT 1 CUP MILLET FLAKES
80G/2¾OZ/SCANT 1 CUP BUCKWHEAT FLAKES
30G/1OZ/SCANT ¼ CUP PUMPKIN SEEDS
30G/1OZ/SCANT ¼ CUP SESAME SEEDS

Preheat the oven to 180°C/350°F/gas 4. Mix together the flakes and seeds in a deep oven dish and roast in the oven for 15–20 minutes until golden brown. Stir every 5 minutes so that the seeds don't burn. Tip out on to a plate to cool, then store in a paper bag in a cool, dry place until needed.

 TOASTED FLAKE PORRIDGE – SERVES 1

40G/1½OZ/HEAPED ⅓ CUP TOASTED FLAKES (SEE ABOVE)
250ML/9FL OZ/GENEROUS 1 CUP MILK OR WATER
½ TSP SALT
GOOSEBERRY JAM AND AN OAT DRINK, YOGURT OR MILK, TO SERVE

Mix the toasted flakes with the milk or water and salt in a heavy-based pan. Bring to the boil, then simmer the porridge for 3 minutes until thick, stirring constantly.

Serve with gooseberry jam and an oat drink, yogurt or milk.

DOCTOR W'S HEALTHY PORRIDGE

This is a recipe that I was given by one of the earliest fibre researchers. In the original recipe, soya milk was used, but this can be replaced with standard low-fat milk. You make a big batch of the porridge, cool it down and store it in the fridge. In the morning, you then only need to warm up a portion in the microwave, but I think it is even easier to cook the porridge in a standard pan. It keeps fresh for four days in the fridge and one portion gives you 14g of dietary fibre! I once ate this porridge with figs soaked in cognac. It wasn't too bad!

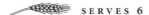 SERVES 6

45G/1¾OZ/⅓ CUP PRUNES
45G/1¾OZ/⅓ CUP RAISINS
350ML/12FL OZ/1½ CUPS WATER
1 LITRE/1¾ PINTS/4⅓ CUPS SOYA MILK (1.5% FAT) OR MILK
1 TBSP GROUND CINNAMON OR COCOA POWDER
80G/2¾OZ/SCANT 1 CUP WHEAT BRAN
70G/2½OZ/¾ CUP OAT BRAN
60G/2¼OZ/¾ CUP ROLLED OATS
60G/2¼OZ/¾ CUP SPROUTING WHEAT
45G/1¾OZ/⅓ CUP WHOLE LINSEEDS
BERRIES, JAM OR FRUIT AND MILK, TO SERVE

Chop the prunes into pieces the size of raisins. Mix together the prunes, raisins, water and soya milk or milk in a pan that holds at least 3 litres/5¼pints/14¼ cups. Bring to the boil. Add the ground cinnamon or cocoa powder. Add the wheat bran, oat bran, rolled oats, sprouting wheat and linseeds. Boil the porridge for at least 3 minutes, or until it has thickened, stirring continuously.

Serve with berries, jam or fruit and milk.

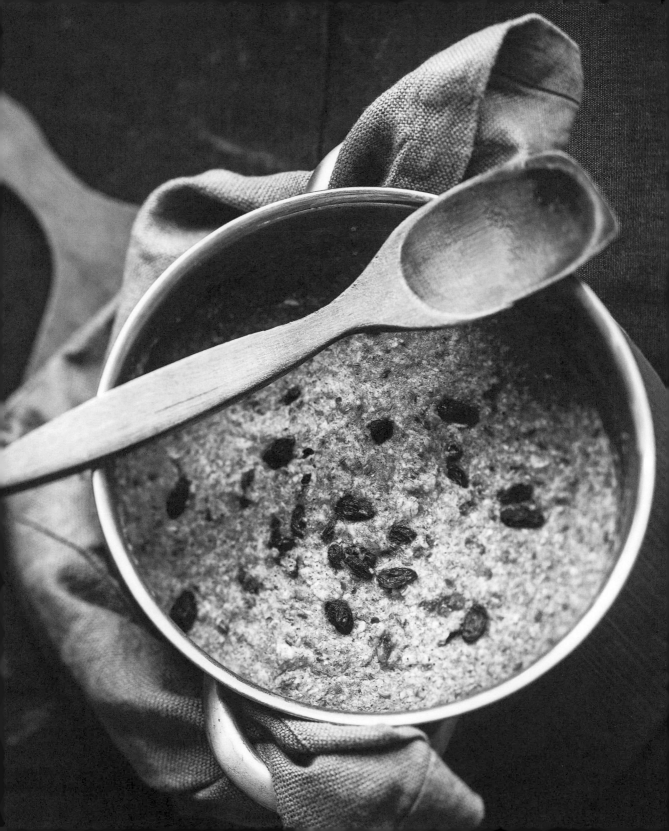

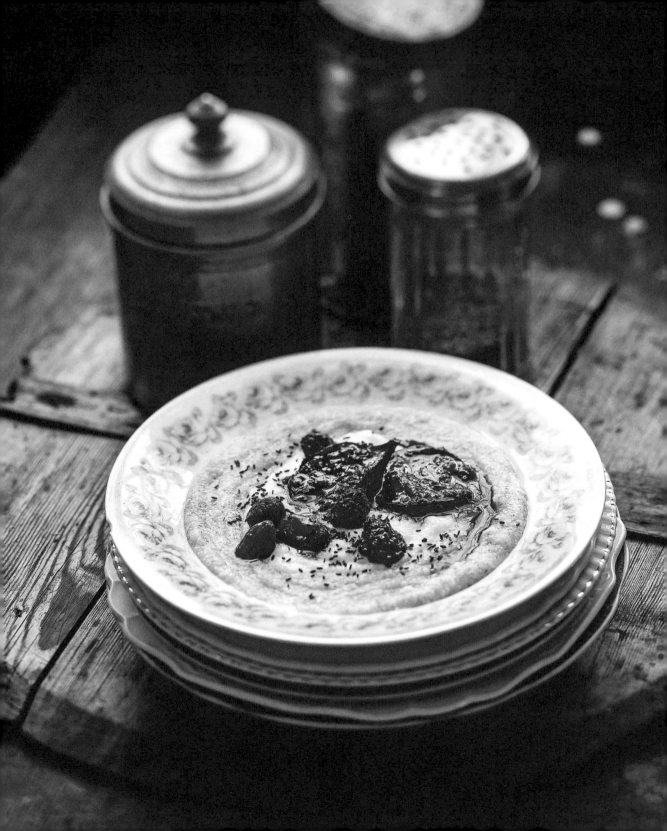

BROWN AND WHITE PORRIDGE

When semolina porridge is combined with porridge made from wholemeal wheat grits, the dietary fibre and wholemeal content increase. With the addition of psyllium seeds and fruit, the fibre content is even greater.

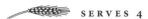 **SERVES 4**

2 PORTIONS OF SEMOLINA PORRIDGE (SEE PAGE 34)
2 PORTIONS OF WHOLEMEAL WHEAT PORRIDGE (SEE PAGE 36)
CHOPPED FRUIT AND PSYLLIUM SEEDS, TO SERVE

Cook the semolina porridge and wheat porridge according to the recipes.

Serve a mixture of the porridges topped with chopped fruit and psyllium seeds.

BLACK AND WHITE PORRIDGE

Serving a mini porridge buffet means that everyone can chose their favourite porridge or a combination of different types of porridge. Vary the buffet with porridge made from grits, flour and flakes so everyone can find new texture and flavour sensations.

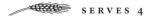 **SERVES 4**

2 PORTIONS SEMOLINA PORRIDGE (SEE PAGE 34)
2 PORTIONS RYE FLOUR PORRIDGE (SEE PAGE 28)
BLUEBERRY HONEY AND DRIED BLUEBERRIES, TO SERVE

Cook the semolina porridge and rye flour porridge according to the recipes.

Serve a mixture of the two porridges together with blueberry honey and dried blueberries.

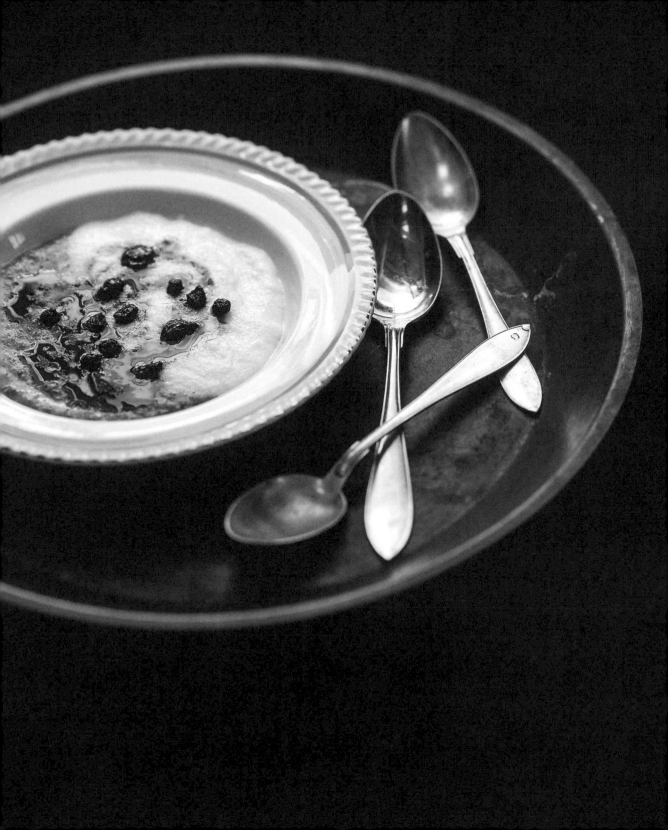

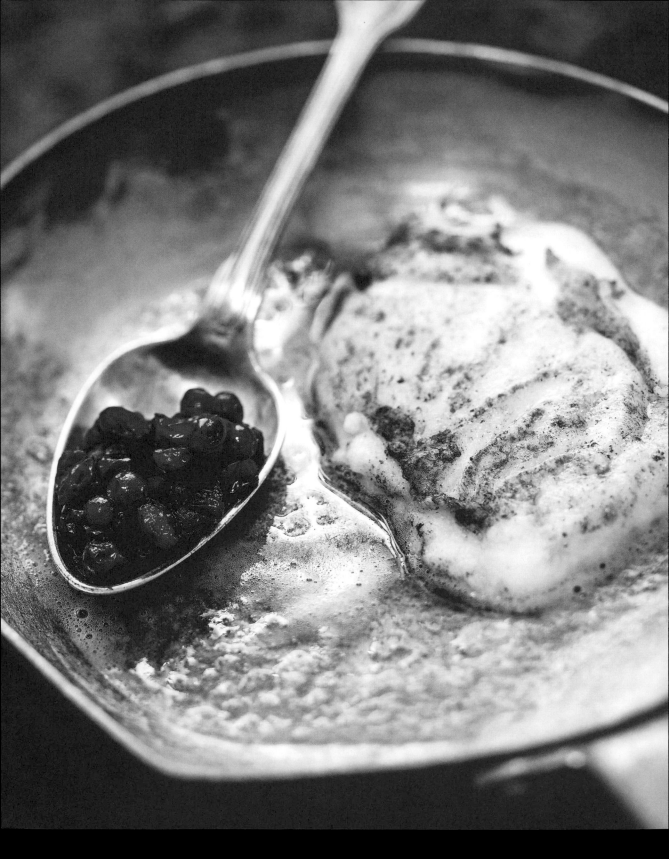

FRIED PORRIDGE

Fried porridge has a lower GI than standard boiled porridge since part of the starch becomes resistant once the porridge has cooled down. The resistant starch has the same qualities as soluble dietary fibre once digested. In the large intestine, short-chain fatty acids, among other things, are produced when the bacteria are feasting on their favourite food-resistant starch. A healthy gut is closely linked to good overall health. Besides, fried porridge tastes great! I made this version with fried Semolina Porridge (see page 34) and traditionally it is served with lingonberries.

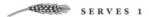 **SERVES 1**

ABOUT 200G/7OZ/SCANT 1 CUP COOKED AND COOLED PORRIDGE (ANY RECIPE)
BUTTER OR MARGARINE, FOR FRYING
SUGAR, CRANBERRIES OR REDCURRANTS AND YOGURT, TO SERVE

Cut the cold porridge into slices. Heat the butter or margarine in a frying pan, add the porridge slices and fry until the porridge has a golden crust and is heated all the way through.

Sprinkle the fried porridge with a little sugar and serve with cranberries or redcurrants and yogurt. Milk is good with it, too!

WHISKED PORRIDGE

This beautiful pink whisked porridge is just as much a dessert as it is a breakfast porridge.

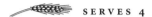 **SERVES 4**

500ML/17FL OZ/GENEROUS 2 CUPS WATER
80G/2¾OZ/¾ CUP CRANBERRY OR REDCURRANT JAM
50G/1¾OZ/HEAPED ⅓ CUP SEMOLINA
COLD MILK, TO SERVE

Put the water and jam in a saucepan and bring to the boil, stirring to mix them together. Whisk in the semolina and leave to simmer for about 5 minutes, stirring constantly. Now it's time for the whipping! Use an electric whisk and whisk until the porridge is light, pink and fluffy.

Serve the porridge lukewarm or cold with cold milk.

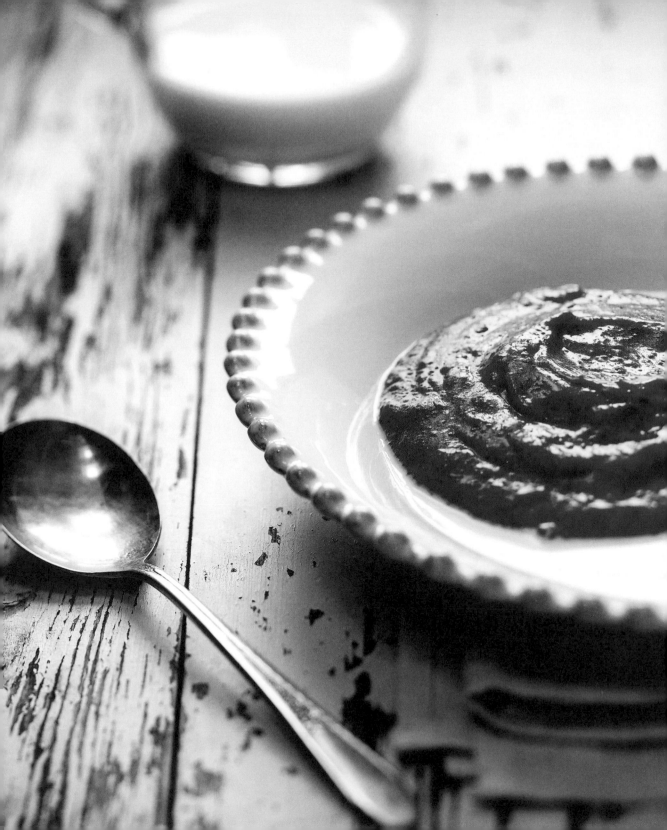

FINNISH POTATO PORRIDGE

There are several old recipes for cooking porridge from potato and flour. In Järvsö, Hälsingland, it is traditional to cook pärgröt, *as it is called, with wheat flour and serve it with pork. This is a Finnish recipe in which the potato porridge is boiled with rye or barley flour and served with milk, a knob of butter and some nice, sharply flavoured jam.*

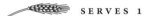 SERVES 1

3 SMALL POTATOES
250ML/9FL OZ/GENEROUS 1 CUP WATER
½ TSP SALT
3 TBSP RYE OR BARLEY FLOUR
A KNOB OF BUTTER
REDCURRANT OR CRANBERRY JAM AND MILK, TO SERVE

Peel and chop the potatoes. Bring the water to the boil in a heavy-based pan. Add the potatoes (the water should just cover the potatoes) and salt, cover and boil until the potato has softened. Drain off and reserve the cooking water. Mash the potato until smooth, diluting it with some of the cooking water, as necessary.

Return the pan to the heat and bring the mixture to the boil, stirring continuously. Still stirring, turn the heat down to low and sift the barley or rye flour over the mash. Continue to simmer for 10–15 minutes, stirring occasionally.

Pop a piece of butter in the middle of the porridge and allow it to melt. Serve with redcurrant or cranberry jam and milk.

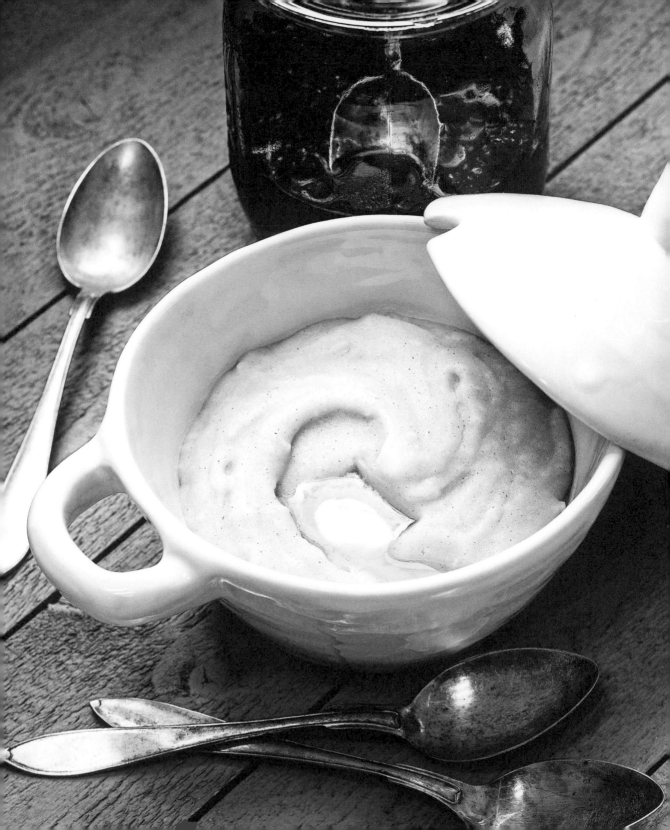

MILLET PORRIDGE

Since millet grains have a bitter coating, the seeds should first be boiled in water that is then discarded. Those who like bitter tastes will like millet porridge as some of this flavour remains in the finished dish. Millet is gluten-free.

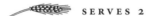 SERVES 2

100G/3½OZ/½ CUP WHOLE MILLET GRAINS
200ML/7FL OZ/SCANT 1 CUP WATER
100G/3½OZ/1 CUP MILLET FLAKES
½–1 PINCH OF SALT
CLEAR HONEY AND MILK, TO SERVE

Bring the millet grains and half the water to the boil, then strain the water off immediately and rinse the millet in cold water.

Mix together the millet grains, millet flakes, salt and the remaining water in a heavy-based pan. Bring to the boil, then simmer the porridge while stirring constantly for 10 minutes. Dilute with more water if needed during the cooking until you have a good porridge consistency.

Serve with clear honey and milk.

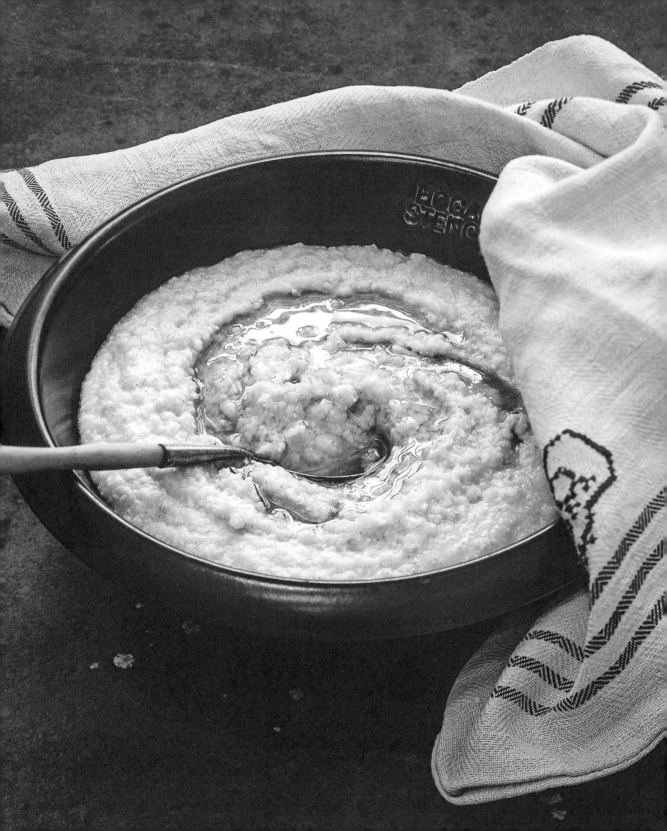

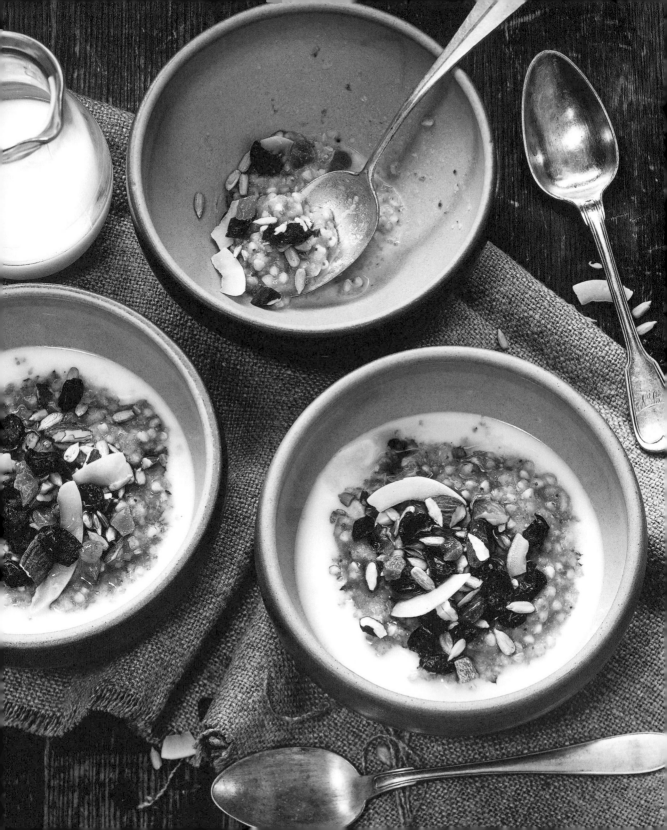

BUCKWHEAT PORRIDGE

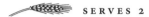 SERVES 2

70G/2½OZ/SCANT ½ CUP BUCKWHEAT GRAINS
450ML/16FL OZ/2 CUPS WATER
40G/1½OZ/HEAPED ⅓ CUP BUCKWHEAT FLAKES
½–1 PINCH OF SALT
DRIED CRANBERRIES, PRUNES, ALMONDS, SUNFLOWER SEEDS, DESICCATED COCONUT, YOGURT
    AND MAPLE SYRUP, TO SERVE

Put the buckwheat grains in a pan with 200ml/7fl oz/scant 1 cup of the water. Bring to the boil, then strain the water off immediately. Add the remaining water, the buckwheat flakes and salt. Return to the boil, then cover and simmer over a low heat for about 10 minutes, stirring occasionally. Turn off the heat and allow the residual heat to cook the porridge for another 10 minutes.

Sprinkle a mixture of dried fruits, nuts and seeds over the top. Drizzle with yogurt and maple syrup to serve.

LINSEED PORRIDGE WITH PRUNES

This is a soothing porridge, ideal for upset stomachs.

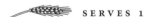 SERVES 1

4 PRUNES
200ML/7FL OZ/SCANT 1 CUP WATER
2 TBSP LINSEEDS
YOGURT AND JAM, TO SERVE

Put the prunes and water in a pan and bring to the boil. Cover and simmer over a low heat until the prunes have softened. Add the linseeds and continue to simmer over a low heat for about 10 minutes until it has turned into porridge.

Serve with yogurt and jam.

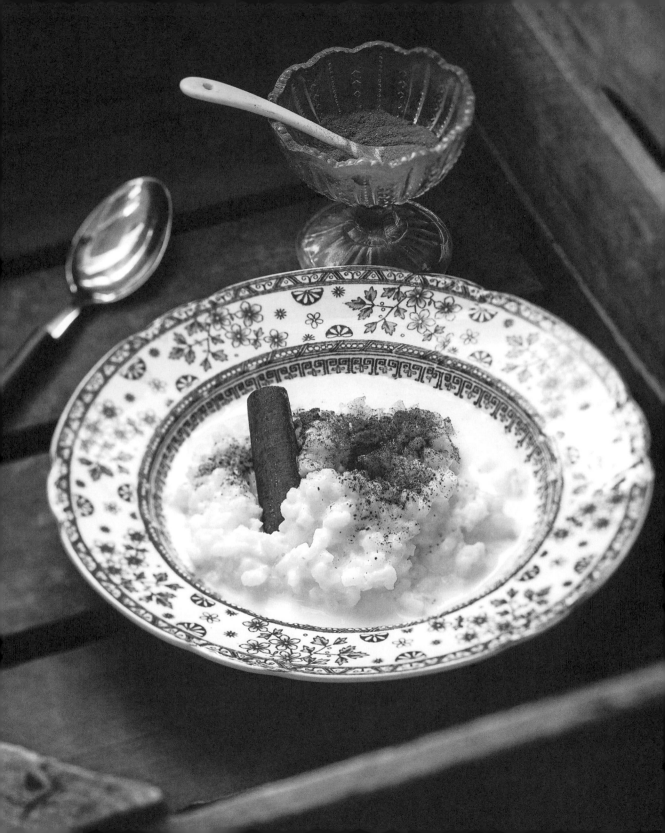

CLASSIC CHRISTMAS PORRIDGE

Porridge made from milk and rice grains began to replace barley porridge and rye porridge at special occasions among the peasantry during the 18th century, and Christmas was such an occasion. Classic Christmas porridge is nowadays eaten all year round. Cinnamon and sugar are associated with Christmas but try fresh berries or strawberry jam as toppings for a different character.

 MAKES 960G/2LB 2OZ/4 CUPS

120G/4¼OZ/⅔ CUP SHORT-GRAIN RICE
300ML/½ PINT/GENEROUS 1¼ CUPS WATER
½ TBSP BUTTER OR MARGARINE
½ TSP SALT
ABOUT 600ML/1 PINT/GENEROUS 2½ CUPS WHOLE MILK, PLUS EXTRA IF NEEDED
GROUND CINNAMON, SUGAR AND MILK, TO SERVE

Mix together the rice, water, butter or margarine and salt in a heavy-based non-stick pan that holds at least 1.5 litres/2½ pints/6½ cups water. Bring to the boil, stirring continuously, then lower the heat and simmer for 10 minutes, stirring occasionally. Add the milk and bring to the boil, stirring all the time, then leave to simmer for about 5 minutes, stirring occasionally.

The first method of finishing this dish is to lower the heat on the hob, cover and leave the porridge to finish cooking for about 30 minutes, stirring regularly.

Alternatively, turn off the heat, cover and leave the porridge to finish cooking in the residual heat for about 45 minutes. Bring the porridge to the boil again. Dilute with more milk if the porridge is too thick. If it is too runny, simmer uncovered, stirring thoroughly, until you have got a good consistency.

Sprinkle with cinnamon and sugar and serve with milk.

Tip Sprinkle the porridge with cinnamon first and then with sugar to avoid the cinnamon floating onto the surface of the milk.

PORRIDGE 'ON THE GO'

This recipe uses Christmas Porridge with Wholemeal Grits as a base but is cooked with a vanilla pod for extra flavour.

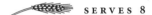 **SERVES 8**

1 VANILLA POD
1 BATCH CHRISTMAS PORRIDGE WITH WHOLEMEAL GRITS (SEE PAGE 18)
150G/5½OZ/⅔ CUP GREEK YOGURT
1–1½ TBSP SUGAR
STRAWBERRY JAM AND FRESH STRAWBERRIES, TO SERVE

Cut the vanilla pod open and scrape out the seeds. Make the porridge according to the recipe on page 18, adding the vanilla seeds and pod at the beginning. Remove the vanilla pod when the porridge is cooked, then leave the porridge to cool.

Mix the cold porridge with the Greek yogurt and sugar. Top with strawberry jam and fresh strawberries, halved or sliced if large, to serve.

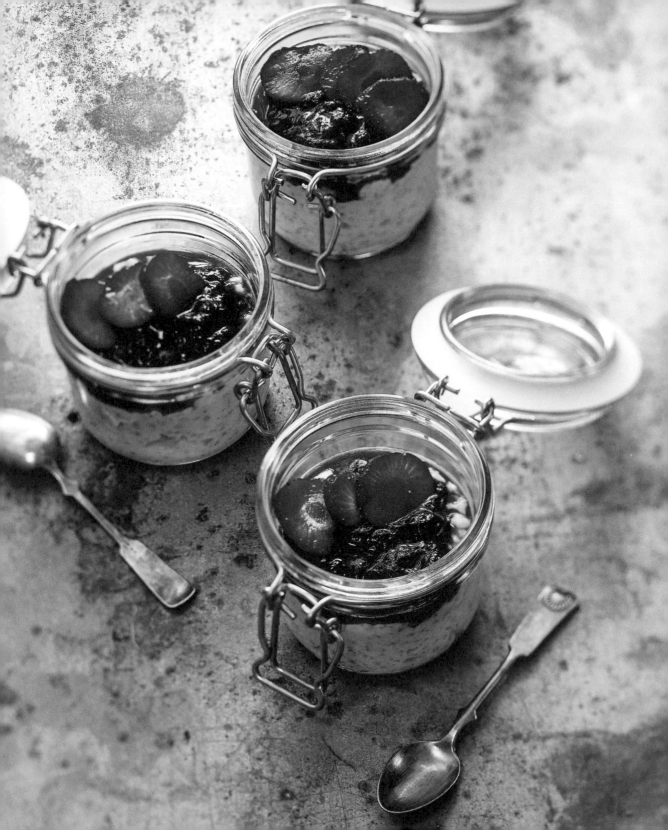

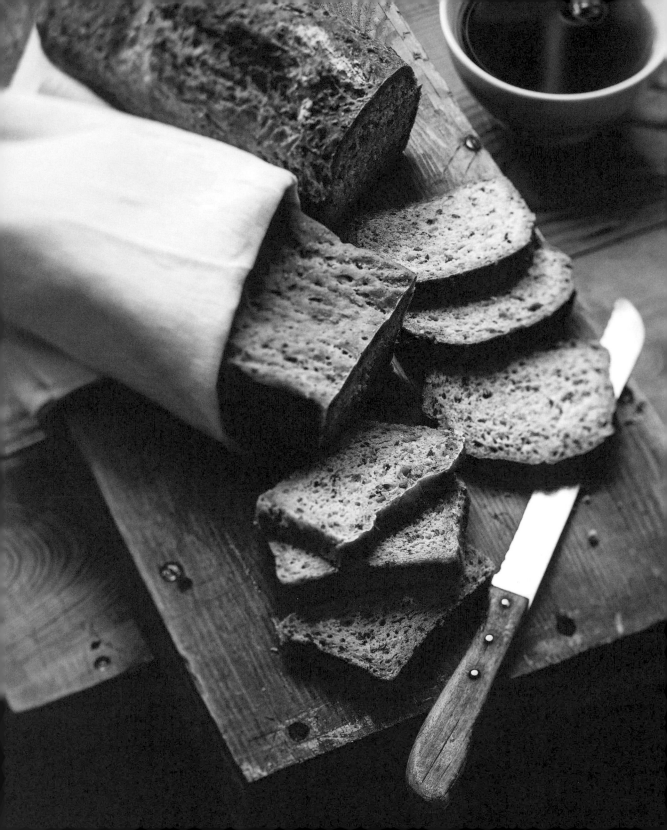

PORRIDGE BREAD

Adding cooked porridge to a bread dough results in a lovely moist loaf. Just be careful when you add the flour as the quantity needed will vary depending on the thickness of the porridge. If you want to use dried yeast, see the tip on page 78.

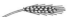 **MAKES 2 X 500G/1LB 2OZ LOAVES**

25G/1 OZ FRESH YEAST

500ML/17FL OZ/GENEROUS 2 CUPS WATER AT 37°C/98°F

2 TBSP RAPESEED OIL

300G/10½OZ/3 CUPS COOKED PORRIDGE

2 TBSP LINSEEDS

1 TSP SALT

2 TSP ANISEEDS

2 TSP FENNEL SEEDS

50G/1¾OZ/HEAPED ⅓ CUP RYE FLOUR

200G/7OZ/⅔ CUP SPELT FLAKES

400G/14OZ/HEAPED 3 CUPS PLAIN FLOUR

Dissolve the yeast in the lukewarm water in a mixing bowl. Add the rapeseed oil, porridge, linseeds, salt, aniseeds and fennel seeds and mix well. Add the rye flour, spelt flakes and then gradually add the plain flour until you have a workable dough. Knead the dough using a dough mixer for 5–10 minutes (or 15–20 minutes by hand) until you have a smooth dough. Cover with oiled clingfilm and leave the dough to rise for 2 hours.

Grease 2 small loaf tins and shape the dough directly into the tins. The dough should be fairly sticky. Leave to rise for 30 minutes.

Preheat the oven to 200°C/400°F/gas 6.

Bake the loaves for about 30 minutes until the temperature in the centre of the loaf is 96°C /204°F or the base of the loaves sound hollow when tapped.

MOTHER MARTA'S PORRIDGE BREAD

If you have a digital probe thermometer, you can check that the bread is ready when the inside temperature has reached 96°C/204°F. If you already have some cooked porridge, you can substitute 400g/14oz/4 cups of cooked porridge for the rolled oats, water and salt. If you want to use dried yeast, see the tip on page 78.

 MAKES 2 X 500G/1LB 2OZ LOAVES

80G/2¾OZ/SCANT 1 CUP ROLLED OATS
400ML/14FL OZ/1¾ CUPS WATER
½ TSP SALT
3½ TBSP RAPESEED OIL
100ML/3½FL OZ/SCANT ½ CUP MILK
30G/1OZ/SCANT ¼ CUP LINSEEDS
25G/1OZ FRESH YEAST
1 TSP GROUND FENNEL SEEDS
½ TSP GROUND ANISEEDS
½ TSP GROUND CARAWAY
200G/7OZ/1⅔ CUPS RYE FLOUR, SIFTED
300G/10½OZ/2½ CUPS PLAIN FLOUR

If you don't have any porridge leftovers, cook the porridge from the rolled oats, water and salt. Remove from the heat and add the oil, milk and linseeds, then leave to cool to 37°C/98°F.

Crumble the yeast into a bowl or directly into the bowl of your dough mixer, add the porridge mixture and spices, and mix thoroughly. Mix the flours together, add 450g/1lb/heaped 3 cups to the porridge mixture and work into a fairly loose dough, adding more flour as needed. Cover with oiled clingfilm and leave to rise for 1 hour.

Grease 2 loaf tins. Work the dough until smooth, then spoon directly into the loaf tins. Cover again and leave to rise for 30 minutes.

Preheat the oven to 200°C/400°F/gas 6.

Bake for about 30 minutes until the loaves reach 94°C/204°F or sound hollow when tapped on the base.

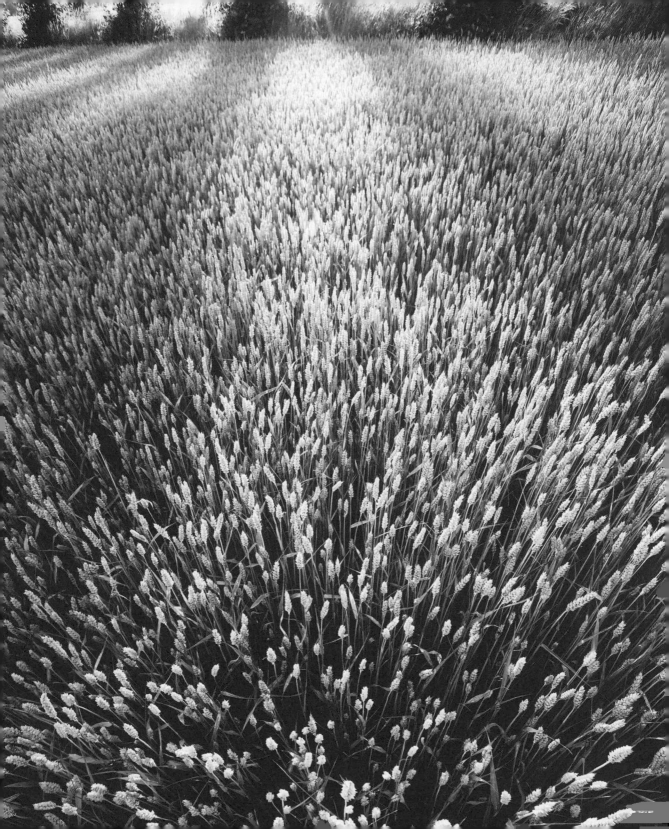

EASY SOFT-CRUST PORRIDGE ROLLS

Wholemeal, linseeds and rapeseed oil will increase both the carbohydrate and fat quality in the bread. If you want to use dried yeast, see the tip below.

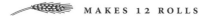 **MAKES 12 ROLLS**

25G/1OZ FRESH YEAST
200ML/7FL OZ/SCANT 1 CUP WATER
100G/3½OZ/ OAT PORRIDGE
1 TBSP RAPESEED OIL
½ TSP SALT
75G/2½OZ/½ CUP RYE FLOUR, SIFTED
90G/3½OZ/SCANT ⅔ CUP BARLEY FLOUR, SIFTED
200G/7OZ/1⅔ CUPS PLAIN FLOUR
2 TBSP LINSEEDS
2 TBSP RYE FLAKES

Dissolve the yeast in the water. Stir in the porridge, rapeseed oil and salt. Mix the flours together and add 300g/10½oz/2¼ cups to the bowl. Work the mixture into a dough and knead for at least 5 minutes. Cover with oiled clingfilm and leave to rise until doubled in size, about 30 minutes.

Preheat the oven to 220°C/425°F/gas 7. Knead the dough again, adding more flour if needed. Divide the dough into 12 pieces and shape into rolls. Mix together the linseeds and rye flakes. Brush the dough balls with cold water, then dip them into the dry mixture. Cover again and leave to rise until the rolls have doubled in size, about 30 minutes. Bake in the oven for about 10 minutes until golden.

Leave the rolls to cool on a rack covered with a tea towel if you want a soft crust.

Tip To use dried yeast instead of fresh, simply substitute 2½ tsp dried yeast for the fresh yeast. To use fast-action dried yeast, mix 1½ tsp with the dry ingredients before mixing in the liquid.

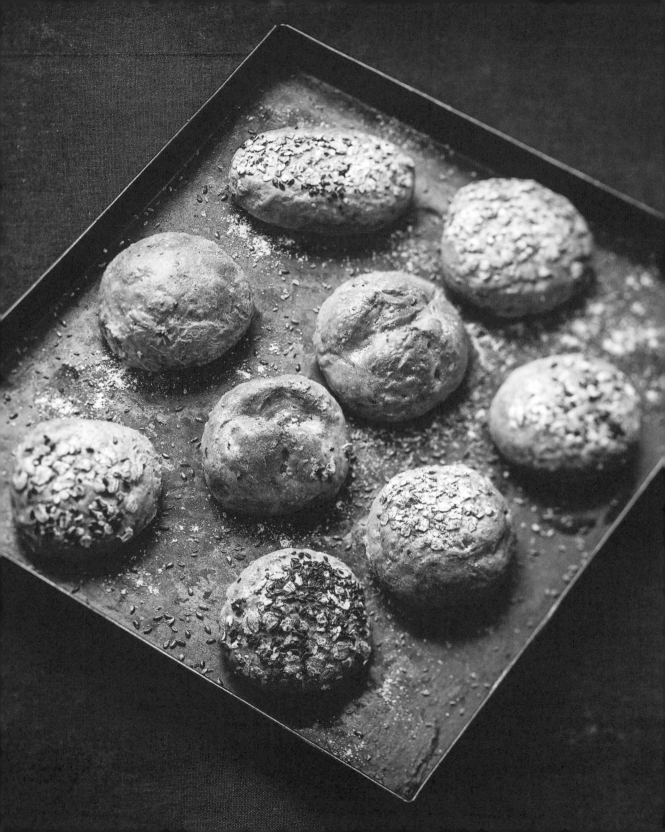

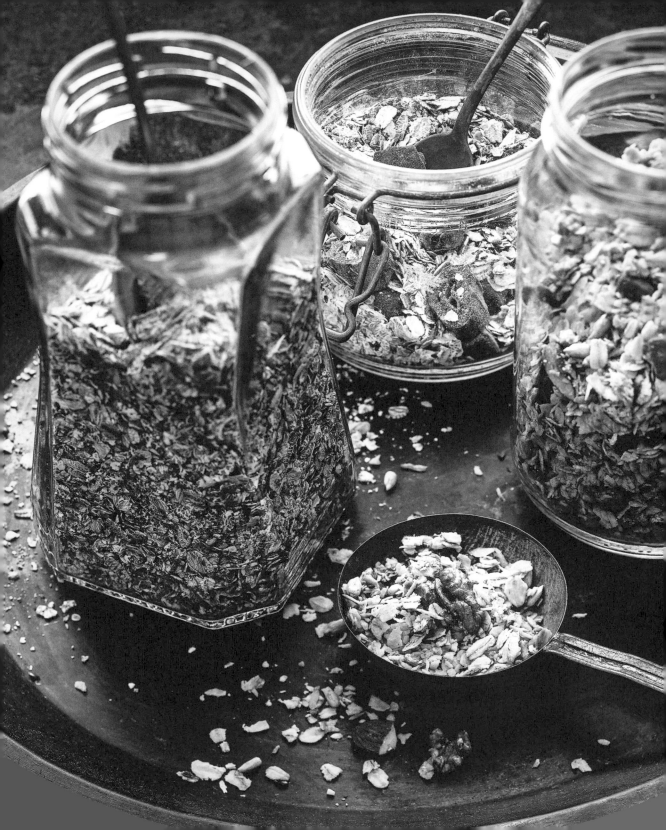

GRANOLA WITH BERRIES AND NUTS

Granola is made from grains toasted with other ingredients to enhance the flavours. In this recipe, the oats are toasted in the oven with oil and honey.

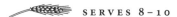 **SERVES 8–10**

60G/2¼OZ/SCANT ½ CUP NUTS, SUCH AS ALMONDS, PECAN NUTS, HAZELNUTS
250G/9OZ/2½ CUPS ROLLED OATS
30G/1OZ/SCANT ½ CUP DESICCATED COCONUT
60G/2¼OZ/SCANT ½ CUP SUNFLOWER SEEDS
30G/1OZ/SCANT ¼ CUP LINSEEDS
4 TBSP RAPESEED OR SUNFLOWER OIL
4 TBSP CLEAR HONEY
80G/2¾OZ/HEAPED ¾ CUP DRIED CHERRIES, DATES, CRANBERRIES OR BLUEBERRIES

Preheat the oven to 180°C/350°F/gas 4.

Coarsely chop the nuts and place in a large bowl with oats, coconut and seeds. Drizzle over the oil and honey and mix thoroughly. Spread the mixture in an even layer in a deep oven dish.

Toast in the oven for about 10 minutes or until the oats have turned golden brown and crisp. Stir occasionally so that you get an even toasting. Take out of the oven and leave to cool.

Stir in the dried fruits and store in an airtight container.

TOASTED BASIC MUESLI

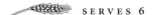 **SERVES 6**

80G/2¾OZ/SCANT 1 CUP ROLLED OATS
80G/2¾OZ/SCANT 1 CUP RYE FLAKES
80G/2¾OZ/SCANT 1 CUP SPELT FLAKES

Preheat the oven to 200°C/400°F/gas 6. Spread out the oats and flakes on a baking sheet. Toast in the oven for about 10 minutes, stirring halfway through. Take out of the oven and leave to cool.

Mix together with different fruits, berries, almonds or nuts according to the suggestions below.

MUESLI MELBA

1 BATCH OF TOASTED BASIC MUESLI (SEE ABOVE)
30G/1OZ/¼ CUP DRIED PEACHES, CHOPPED
30G/1OZ/¼ CUP DRIED RASPBERRIES

BLUEBERRY AND RASPBERRY MUESLI

1 BATCH OF TOASTED BASIC MUESLI (SEE ABOVE)
30G/1OZ/¼ CUP DRIED BLUEBERRIES
30G/1OZ/¼ CUP DRIED RASPBERRIES

ALMOND MUESLI

1 BATCH OF TOASTED BASIC MUESLI (SEE ABOVE)
30G/1OZ/¼ CUP ALMONDS OR OTHER NUTS

RAW MUESLI WITH DATES

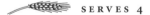 **SERVES 4**

40G/1½OZ/SCANT ½ CUP ROLLED OATS
40G/1½OZ/SCANT ½ CUP RYE FLAKES
40G/1½OZ/SCANT ½ CUP SPELT FLAKES
1 TBSP ROSEHIP FLOUR
2 TBSP PSYLLIUM SEEDS
½ TBSP SUGAR (OPTIONAL)
120G/4½OZ/SCANT 1 CUP CHOPPED PITTED DATES

In a jar, mix together the oats, rye and spelt flakes, rosehip flour, psyllium seeds, sugar, if using, and dates. If you are using soft dates, be careful not to make a batch that is too big as it can go mouldy. It will keep fresh for about a week.

CRISPBREAD MUESLI

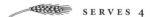 **SERVES 4**

4 SLICES OAT CRISPBREAD
4 SLICES RYE CRISPBREAD
MILK OR YOGURT
FRESH BERRIES, FRUIT OR JAM, TO SERVE

Crumble the crispbread directly into milk or yogurt. Add fresh berries, fruit or jam to serve.

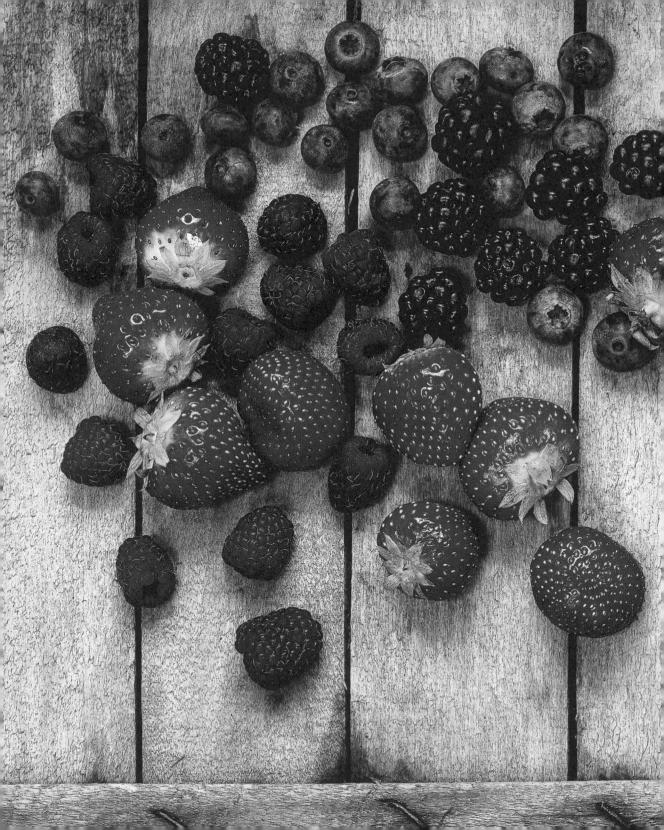

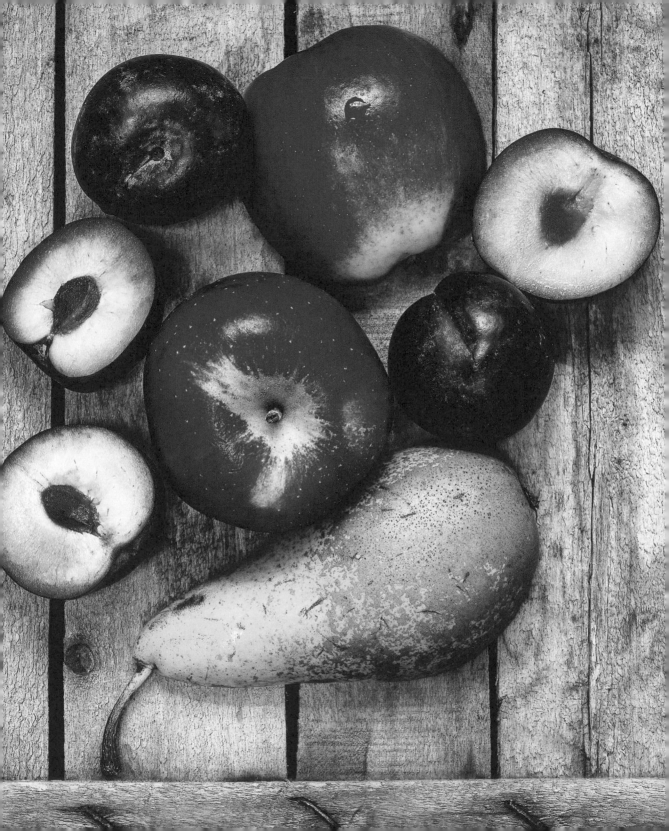

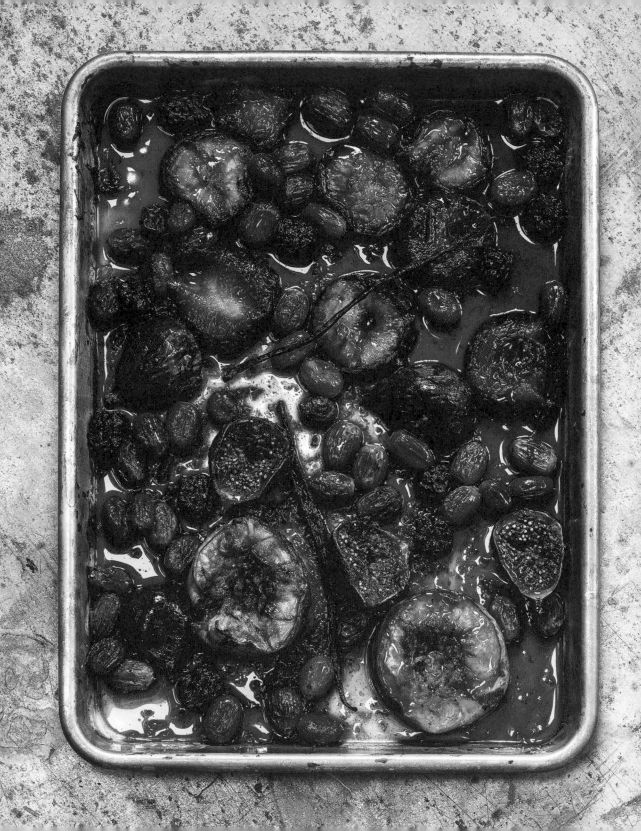

BAKED FRUIT

Baked fruit is delicious served with porridge. It will keep for several days in the fridge in an airtight container but it is best served freshly made or at room temperature. Use fruits in season so substitute suitable choices, if necessary, with those listed below.

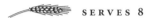 **SERVES 8**

4 PLUMS

1–2 NECTARINES

2 FIGS

55G/2OZ/SCANT ½ CUP FROZEN OR FRESH BLACKBERRIES

65G/2½OZ/SCANT ½ CUP GRAPES

FOR THE DRESSING

FINELY GRATED ZEST AND JUICE OF 1 ORGANIC ORANGE

1 VANILLA POD, CUT OPEN AND SEEDS SCRAPED OUT

3 TBSP SUGAR

Preheat the oven to 200°C/400°F/gas 6. Halve the plums and the nectarines and remove the stones. Cut the figs in half and place all the fruit in one layer in a large oven dish with the rounded sides facing up. Sprinkle over the blackberries and grapes.

Mix together the zest and juice from the orange with the seeds from the vanilla pod and the sugar. Pour over the fruit in the dish. Add the scraped-out vanilla pod. Bake in the oven for about 45–50 minutes until the fruit has softened. Serve warm or cold with your favourite porridge.

Tip If you cannot get hold of the fruit above you can try sliced apples, orange slices or other seasonal fruit.

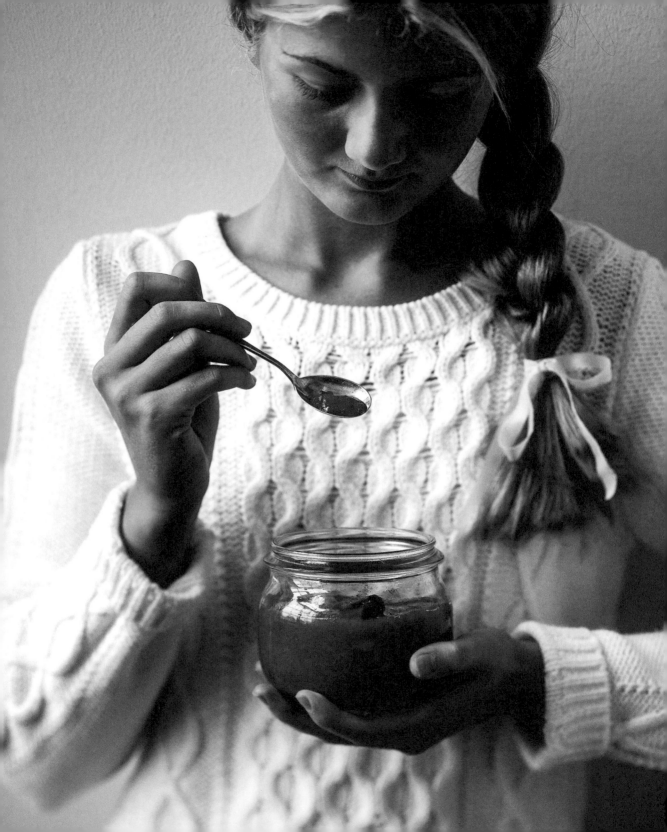

STRAWBERRY AND RHUBARB COMPÔTE

Compôte makes a luxurious porridge topping.

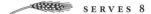 **SERVES 8**

300G/10½OZ RHUBARB
200G/7OZ/1¼ CUPS STRAWBERRIES
80G/2¾OZ/SCANT ½ CUP DEMERARA SUGAR
1 CINNAMON STICK

Slice the rhubarb and cut the strawberries into smaller pieces. Place everything in a wide pan and add the sugar and cinnamon stick. Bring to the boil, then leave to simmer in its own juice over a low heat for about 20 minutes until you get a thick compôte.

Serve warm or cold with your porridge.

GOOSEBERRY JAM

Gooseberries are rich in bioactive tannins and the capacity to fight off acid radicals is 17 times higher in gooseberries than in pomegranate.

 MAKES ABOUT 750ML/26FL OZ JAM

650G/1LB 7OZ/10 CUPS FRESH GOOSEBERRIES, TOPPED AND TAILED
300ML/½ PINT/1¼ CUPS WATER
1 TSP COARSELY CRUSHED CARDAMOM SEEDS
375G/13OZ/SCANT 2¼ CUPS SUGAR
1½ TBSP GRATED FRESH ROOT GINGER

Top and tail the gooseberries and put in a pan with the water. Bring to the boil, cover and simmer for 15 minutes. Remove the pan from the heat. Stir in the cardamom and sugar, a little at a time, until dissolved. Return the pan to the heat and leave to simmer, stirring constantly, for about 10 minutes until the jam has set.

Remove the pan from the heat and skim thoroughly. Stir in the ginger. The jam should not be boiled after you have added the ginger. Pour into warm sterilized glass jars and seal. Store in a cool place.

FRESH RASPBERRY JAM

In Sweden, this would be made with cloudberries.

 MAKES ABOUT 250G/9OZ JAM

280G/10OZ/2 CUPS RASPBERRIES OR CLOUDBERRIES
75–120G/2½–4¼OZ/SCANT ½–⅔ CUP GRANULATED SUGAR

Stir the berries and sugar together until the sugar has dissolved. Pour into a sterilized jar, seal the lid and store in the fridge.

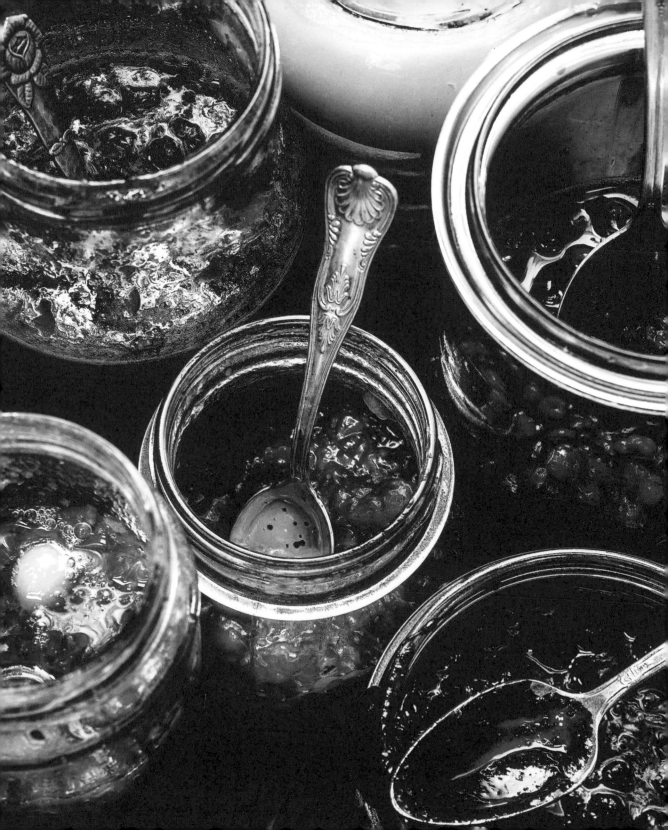

BLUEBERRY JAM

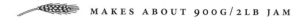 MAKES ABOUT 900G/2LB JAM

500G/1LB 2OZ/4¼ CUPS BLUEBERRIES
200G/7OZ/HEAPED 1 CUP GRANULATED SUGAR
200G/7OZ/HEAPED 1 CUP JAM SUGAR
1 VANILLA POD

Layer the blueberries, granulated sugar and jam sugar in a large pan. Cut open the vanilla pod, scrape out the seeds and add both seeds and pod to the pan. Heat up slowly, stirring continuously, until the sugar has dissolved. Raise the heat and leave the jam to boil for about 15 minutes. Skim thoroughly. Remove the vanilla pod.

Pour the jam into warm sterilized jars and seal. Store the jars in the fridge.

FRESH CRANBERRY JAM

In Sweden, this would be made with lingonberries.

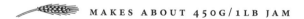 MAKES ABOUT 450G/1LB JAM

500G/1LB 2OZ/4¼ CUPS CRANBERRIES OR LINGONBERRIES
150–300G/5½–10½OZ/¾–1½ CUPS GRANULATED SUGAR
½ CINNAMON STICK

Stir the berries and 150g/5½oz/¾ cup of the sugar together in a heavy-based pan until the sugar has dissolved. Check the flavour and add more sugar if it needs more sweetness. Pour into thoroughly cleaned jars. Add a small chunk of the cinnamon stick to each jar. Seal and store in the fridge.

APPLE SAUCE

This is a great standby to store in the freezer.

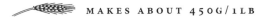 **MAKES ABOUT 450G/1LB**

1KG/2LB 4OZ APPLES
4 TBSP WATER
GRANULATED SUGAR, TO TASTE

Peel the apples and remove the cores. Bring the water to the boil in a pan. Cut the apples into smaller chunks directly into the boiling water. Cover and simmer the apple pieces over a low heat until soft. Mash the apples with a hand-held blender or rub through a sieve. Add sugar to taste.

Since the sauce has no preservatives, it can go off quite quickly so it is best to freeze it. You can freeze it in small jars, leaving a good air space at the top as the sauce expands when frozen, and use whenever you need it.

NUTRITIONAL DATA

The following tables can be used to calculate the nutritional values of a porridge meal.

Vitamins, minerals, fat quality and dietary fibre in porridge toppings
In the below table the nutritional content is shown per tablespoon (tbsp), 100ml (ml) or per item.

Dietary fibre and wholemeal in porridge and muesli
The nutritional values shown in the table opposite are per portion of porridge or muesli according to the recipes in the book, unless otherwise specified. If variations are offered for the cooking liquid, for example water or milk of varying fat content, the table specifies which liquid the nutritional values are based on.

Fat content of whole milk is calculated at 3 percent and of semi-skimmed milk at 1.5 percent.

Vitamins, minerals, fat quality and dietary fibre in porridge toppings	Quantity	Energy (kcal)	Vitamin C (mg)	Iron (mg)	Magnesium (mg)	Potassium (mg)	Saturated fat (g)	Mono-unsaturated fat	Poly-unsaturated fat	Dietary fibre (g)
Almonds	1 tbsp	60	0	0.5	28	73	0.5	3.4	1.1	0.7
Apple	1 medium	65	15	0.2	6	143	0	0	0	2.3
Apricots, dried	65g	109	1	2.9	20	676	0	0.1	0	5.9
Blueberries, fresh	50g/1¾oz/heaped ⅓ cup	28	3	0.4	5	52	0	0.1	0.3	1.9
Blueberry jam	1 tbsp	24	0	0.1	0	8	0	0	0	0.3
Cloudberries, fresh	1 tbsp	4	5	0.1	2	15	0	0	0	0.5
Dates, dried	60g/2¼oz/scant ½ cup	216	0	1	26	488	0	0.1	0.2	4.5
Gooseberries, fresh	1 tbsp	3	3	0	1	13	0	0	0	0.3
Hazelnuts	1 tbsp	58	0	0.3	14	40	0.4	4.4	0.6	0.5
Lingonberries, fresh	1 tbsp	5	0	0	1	8	0	0	0	0.2
Linseeds	1 tbsp	52	0	0	1	8	0	0	0	0.2
Milk (3% fat)	100ml/3½fl oz/scant ½ cup	62	1	0	12	167	2.1	0.7	0.1	0
Milk (5% fat)	100ml/3½fl oz/scant ½ cup	41	1	0	12	173	0.3	0.1	0	0
Pear	1 medium	58	6	0.2	9	132	0	0	0	4.8
Prunes	60g/2¼oz/scant ½ cup	181	2	1.5	40	570	0.1	0	0.2	6.7
Raisins	60g/2¼oz/scant ½ cup	182	2	1.5	18	458	0.1	0	0.1	5.9
Raspberries, fresh	60g/2¼oz/½ cup	15	14	0.1	13	78	0	0	0.2	1.9
Rosehip drink	100ml/3½fl oz/scant ½ cup	48	25	0.2	6	61	0	0	0	0.6
Sugar	1 tbsp	57	0	0	0	0	0	0	0	0
Sunflower seeds	1 tbsp	52	0	0.6	32	62	0.5	0.9	2.9	0.5
Walnuts	1 tbsp	40	0	0.1	9	30	0.3	0.9	2.3	0.3
Yogurt, natural (0.5% fat)	100g/3½oz/scant ½ cup	44	1	0	15	190	0.3	0.1	0	0
Yogurt, natural 3% fat	100g/3½oz/scant ½ cup	62	1	0	12	167	2.1	0.7	0.1	0

Dietary fibre and wholemeal in porridge and muesli (1 portion)	Recipe page	Energy (kcal)	Dietary fibre (g)	Beta-glucan (g)	Wholemeal (g)
Baked Apple Porridge	47	193	3	0.2	7
Barley Porridge with Oats, made with milk (milk 0.5%)	17	169	5	1	23
Barley Porridge with Oats, made with water	17	122	10	1	23
Bircher Muesli	44	213	3	0.2	8
Blueberry and Raspberry Porridge	34	214	3	0	0
Blueberry Porridge, made with semolina (milk 1.5%)	33	255	3	0	0
Blueberry Porridge, made with wholemeal wheat grits (milk 1.5%)	33	247	4	0	18
Buckwheat Porridge	69	246	4	0	0
Christmas Porridge with Wholemeal Grits	18	184	1	0.3	7
Classic Christmas Porridge (milk 3%)	71	224	7	0	0
Crème Fraîche Porridge	33	328	5	0	0
Crispbread Muesli	83	97	5	0	22
Davos Porridge	43	324	5	1	40
Doctor W's Healthy Porridge	54	288	14	1	9
Finnish Potato Porridge	64	167	1	0.5	24
Granola with Berries and Nuts	81	234	1	0.6	18
Linseed Porridge with Prunes	69	150	10	0	0
Millet Porridge	66	209	1	0	60
Oat Bran Porridge	12	129	2	2.9	0
Oat Porridge	8	148	7	1.2	40
Oat Porridge Melba	11	213	4	1.2	40
Oat Porridge with Caramel Coating	8	205	8	1.2	40
Pajala Porridge	50	163	4	0.5	4
Porridge 'On the Go'	72	124	5	0.1	3
Raw Muesli with Dates	83	223	8	0.3	30
Rye Flake Porridge	28	139	5	0	40
Rye Flour Porridge	28	120	1	0	40
Semolina Porridge	34	261	5	0	0
Skier's Porridge	48	141	2	1	40
Toasted Basic Muesli	82	195	7	0.6	60
Toasted Flake Porridge	53	226	4	0.3	40
Toasted Oat Flour Porridge	15	192	1	0.6	25
Wet Muesli	43	534	7	0.8	25
Wheat Flour Porridge	30	223	1	0	0
Wheat Flour Porridge with Butter	30	259	7	0	0
Whisked Porridge	62	155	3	0	0
Wholemeal Wheat Porridge (milk 1.5%)	36	152	3	0	30

Note: The consumption of salt should not exceed 5–6g (about 1 tsp). A pinch of salt added to your porridge contains 0.4mg sodium.

RECIPE INDEX

OAT PORRIDGE

OAT BRAN PORRIDGE 12

OAT PORRIDGE 8

OAT PORRIDGE WITH CARAMEL COATING 8

OAT PORRIDGE MELBA 11

TOASTED OAT FLOUR PORRIDGE 15

BARLEY PORRIDGE

BARLEY PORRIDGE WITH OATS 17

CHRISTMAS PORRIDGE WITH WHOLEMEAL
  GRITS 18

RYE PORRIDGE

RYE FLAKE PORRIDGE 28

RYE FLOUR PORRIDGE 28

WHEAT PORRIDGE

BLUEBERRY PORRIDGE 33

BLUEBERRY AND RASPBERRY PORRIDGE 34

CRÈME FRAÎCHE PORRIDGE 33

SEMOLINA PORRIDGE 34

WHEAT FLOUR PORRIDGE WITH BUTTER 30

WHOLEMEAL WHEAT PORRIDGE 36

DIFFERENT KINDS OF PORRIDGE

BAKED APPLE PORRIDGE 47

BIRCHER MUESLI 44

BLACK AND WHITE PORRIDGE 58

BROWN AND WHITE PORRIDGE 57

BUCKWHEAT PORRIDGE 69

CLASSIC CHRISTMAS PORRIDGE 71

DAVOS PORRIDGE 43

DOCTOR W'S HEALTHY PORRIDGE 54

FINNISH POTATO PORRIDGE 64

FRIED PORRIDGE 61

LINSEED PORRIDGE WITH PRUNES 69

MILLET PORRIDGE 66

PAJALA PORRIDGE 50

PORRIDGE 'ON THE GO' 72

SKIER'S PORRIDGE 48

TOASTED FLAKE PORRIDGE 53

WET MUESLI 43

WHISKED PORRIDGE 62

PORRIDGE BREAD

EASY SOFT-CRUST PORRIDGE ROLLS 78

MOTHER MARTA'S PORRIDGE BREAD 76

PORRIDGE BREAD 75

MUESLI AND GRANOLA

ALMOND MUESLI 82

CRISPBREAD MUESLI 83

GRANOLA WITH BERRIES AND NUTS 81

MUESLI MELBA 82

BLUEBERRY AND RASPBERRY MUESLI 82

RAW MUESLI WITH DATES 83

TOASTED BASIC MUESLI 82

FRUIT AND JAM

APPLE SAUCE 93

BAKED FRUIT 87

BLUEBERRY JAM 92

FRESH CRANBERRY JAM 92

FRESH RASPBERRY JAM 90

GOOSEBERRY JAM 90

STRAWBERRY AND RHUBARB COMPÔTE 89

Viola Adamsson is a Doctor of Medical Science. She has worked as a nutrition manager in the food industry and has also been a dietary advisor to top athletes, including the Swedish national cross-country skiing team. Viola has previously published the Gourmand Cook Book award-winning title, **The Best of Nordic Food**.